JUICING FOR ACID REFLUX RELIEF

By

Jane F Garraway

Copyright © 2024

TABLE OF CONTENT

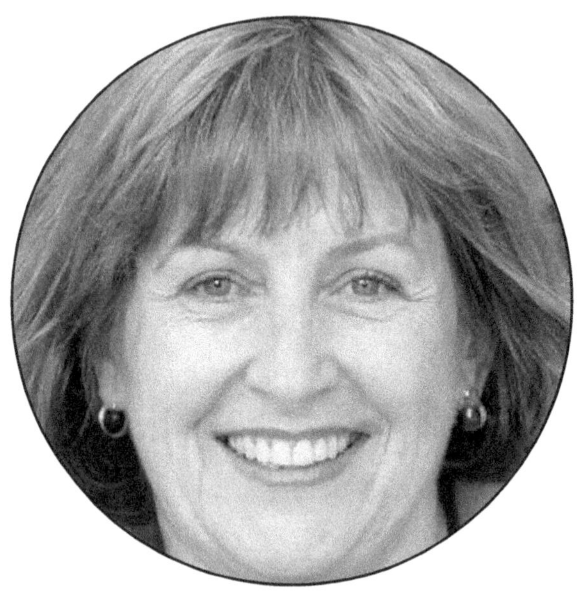

Welcome!

I am thrilled to have you purchase this book. Whether you are an experienced home cook or just starting out, my collection of recipes is always designed to inspire and my goal is to make cooking an enjoyable and healthy experience for everyone.

Within these pages, you'll find a diverse range of juices, each crafted with love and attention to detail.

Cooking is not just about preparing food; it's about creating memories, exploring new flavors, and sharing delicious and healthy meals with your loved ones. I encourage you to experiment, make these recipes your own, and savor every moment of the process.

Thank you for allowing me to be a part of your journey. Let's get cooking!

Jane Garraway

Understanding Acid Reflux: Causes, Symptoms, and Management

Acid reflux, also known as gastroesophageal reflux disease (GERD), is a common digestive disorder that affects millions of individuals worldwide.

Causes of Acid Reflux:

1. **Lower Esophageal Sphincter (LES) Dysfunction:** The LES, a ring-like muscle that separates the stomach from the esophagus, may weaken or relax, allowing stomach acid to flow back into the esophagus.
2. **Hiatal Hernia:** A condition in which a portion of the stomach protrudes into the diaphragm, potentially compromising the LES's function.
3. **Dietary Triggers:** Consuming acidic, spicy, or fatty foods, as well as caffeine, alcohol, and chocolate, can prompt reflux episodes.
4. **Overeating and Large Meals:** A full stomach puts pressure on the LES, increasing the likelihood of acid reflux.
5. **Obesity:** Excess weight, especially around the abdomen, can contribute to LES dysfunction and acid reflux.
6. **Pregnancy:** Hormonal changes and increased pressure on the abdomen during pregnancy can trigger acid reflux.
7. **Smoking:** Nicotine weakens the LES and smoking increases acid production.

Symptoms of Acid Reflux:

1. **Heartburn:** A burning sensation in the chest that may radiate to the throat.
2. **Regurgitation:** Sour or bitter-tasting fluid backing up into the mouth or throat.
3. **Dysphagia:** Difficulty swallowing or a sensation of food getting stuck.
4. **Chronic Cough:** A persistent cough, particularly at night, due to acid irritating the throat.
5. **Hoarseness:** Changes in voice tone or persistent throat clearing.
6. **Chest Pain:** Discomfort that may mimic heart-related pain.
7. **Asthma Exacerbation:** Worsening of asthma symptoms triggered by acid reflux.

Effective Management Strategies

1. **Dietary Modifications:** Avoid trigger foods and beverages, opt for smaller, more frequent meals, and eat slowly.
2. **Lifestyle Changes:** Maintain a healthy weight, avoid smoking, and elevate the head of your bed if symptoms worsen at night.
3. **Meal Timing:** Avoid eating large meals close to bedtime to reduce the risk of nighttime reflux.
4. **Maintain Good Posture:** Sit upright during and after meals to promote proper digestion.
5. **Stay Hydrated:** Drink water throughout the day to help dilute stomach acid.
6. **Chew Gum:** Chewing sugar-free gum after meals can stimulate saliva production, which helps neutralize acid.
7. **Medications:** Over-the-counter antacids or prescribed medications like proton pump inhibitors (PPIs) can provide relief by reducing acid production.
8. **Natural Remedies:** Herbal teas (such as chamomile or ginger), deglycyrrhizinated licorice (DGL), and aloe vera juice may offer soothing effects.
9. **Consult a Healthcare Professional:** If symptoms persist or worsen, consult a healthcare provider for accurate diagnosis and personalized treatment.

By understanding the causes, recognizing symptoms, and implementing effective management strategies, you can take control of your acid reflux and GERD symptoms. Empower yourself with knowledge, make mindful choices, and work closely with healthcare professionals to achieve optimal digestive health and overall well-being.

Navigating Your Diet for Acid Reflux and GERD

Foods to Embrace:

1. **Lean Proteins:** Opt for skinless poultry, fish, and lean cuts of meat to provide essential nutrients without excess fat.
2. **Non-Citrus Fruits:** Enjoy bananas, melons, apples, and pears, which are lower in acidity and less likely to trigger symptoms.
3. **Vegetables:** Most non-starchy veggies, like leafy greens, broccoli, cauliflower, and carrots, are gentle on the stomach.
4. **Whole Grains:** Incorporate whole grains like oats, brown rice, quinoa, and whole wheat bread for a fiber-rich diet.
5. **Low-Fat Dairy:** Choose skim or low-fat dairy products like yogurt and cheese to minimize fat content.
6. **Healthy Fats:** Opt for sources like avocados, nuts, seeds, and olive oil to add flavor and nourishment.
7. **Ginger:** Known for its soothing properties, ginger can be included in teas, dishes, or as a seasoning.
8. **Herbal Teas:** Chamomile, licorice, and mint teas can help soothe the digestive system.

Foods to Approach with Caution:

1. **Citrus Fruits:** While nutritious, citrus fruits like oranges, grapefruits, and lemons can be acidic and trigger symptoms in some individuals.
2. **Tomatoes and Tomato-Based Products:** These can be acidic and may cause discomfort for some people.
3. **Onions and Garlic:** These can relax the LES and contribute to reflux.
4. Spicy Foods: Limit consumption of spicy dishes as they may irritate the esophagus.
5. **Chocolate:** Enjoy chocolate in moderation, as it may relax the LES and worsen symptoms.
6. **Peppermint**: Though soothing, peppermint can relax the LES and lead to reflux.
7. **Carbonated Beverages:** The bubbles can increase pressure on the stomach, potentially causing acid to flow back into the esophagus.

Foods to Avoid:

1. **High-Fat Foods:** Fried foods, full-fat dairy, and fatty cuts of meat can relax the LES and worsen symptoms.
2. **Alcohol:** Alcohol can weaken the LES and increase acid production.
3. **Caffeine:** Limit coffee, tea, and other caffeinated beverages, as they can stimulate acid production.
4. **Mint:** Mint-flavored foods, candies, and gums may exacerbate reflux symptoms.
5. **Spicy Condiments:** Avoid hot sauces, chili pepper, and excessive use of black pepper.

PART ONE

JUICES

Guava Ginger Juice

This refreshing juice is packed with stomach-soothing properties to help alleviate acid reflux symptoms. Made with alkaline-forming guava and anti-inflammatory ginger, it provides a gentle and delicious way to manage discomfort.

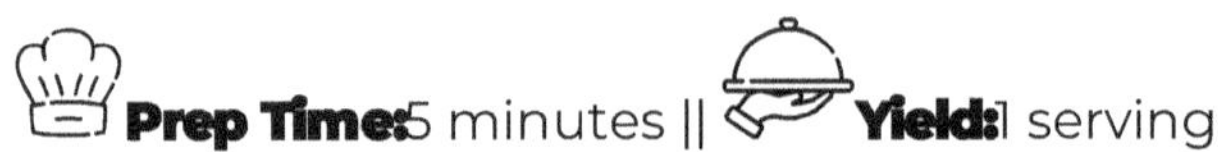
Prep Time: 5 minutes || **Yield:** 1 serving

INGREDIENTS
- 2 ripe guavas, peeled and seeded
- 1 inch knob of ginger, peeled

INSTRUCTIONS
1. Wash the guavas thoroughly and remove the peel with a knife. Cut the guavas in half and remove the seeds.
2. Peel the ginger with a spoon or vegetable peeler.
3. Juice the guavas and ginger together using a juicer.
4. Enjoy the juice immediately for maximum freshness.

NOTES
- You can adjust the amount of ginger depending on your taste preference. Start with a smaller piece and add more if desired.
- If you don't have a juicer, you can blend the ingredients with a little water and then strain the pulp. However, juicing provides a more concentrated dose of nutrients.
- Guavas can vary in sweetness. If your guavas are not very sweet, you can add a splash of apple juice or a squeeze of honey for additional flavor (be mindful if you have severe acid reflux).

EXTRA TIPS
- Drink this juice on an empty stomach, at least 30 minutes before a meal, for optimal relief.
- Avoid acidic fruits like oranges, grapefruits, and pineapples when dealing with acid reflux.
- Consider adding a handful of spinach or kale for a boost of vitamins and minerals, but be aware these can be slightly acidic for some people.

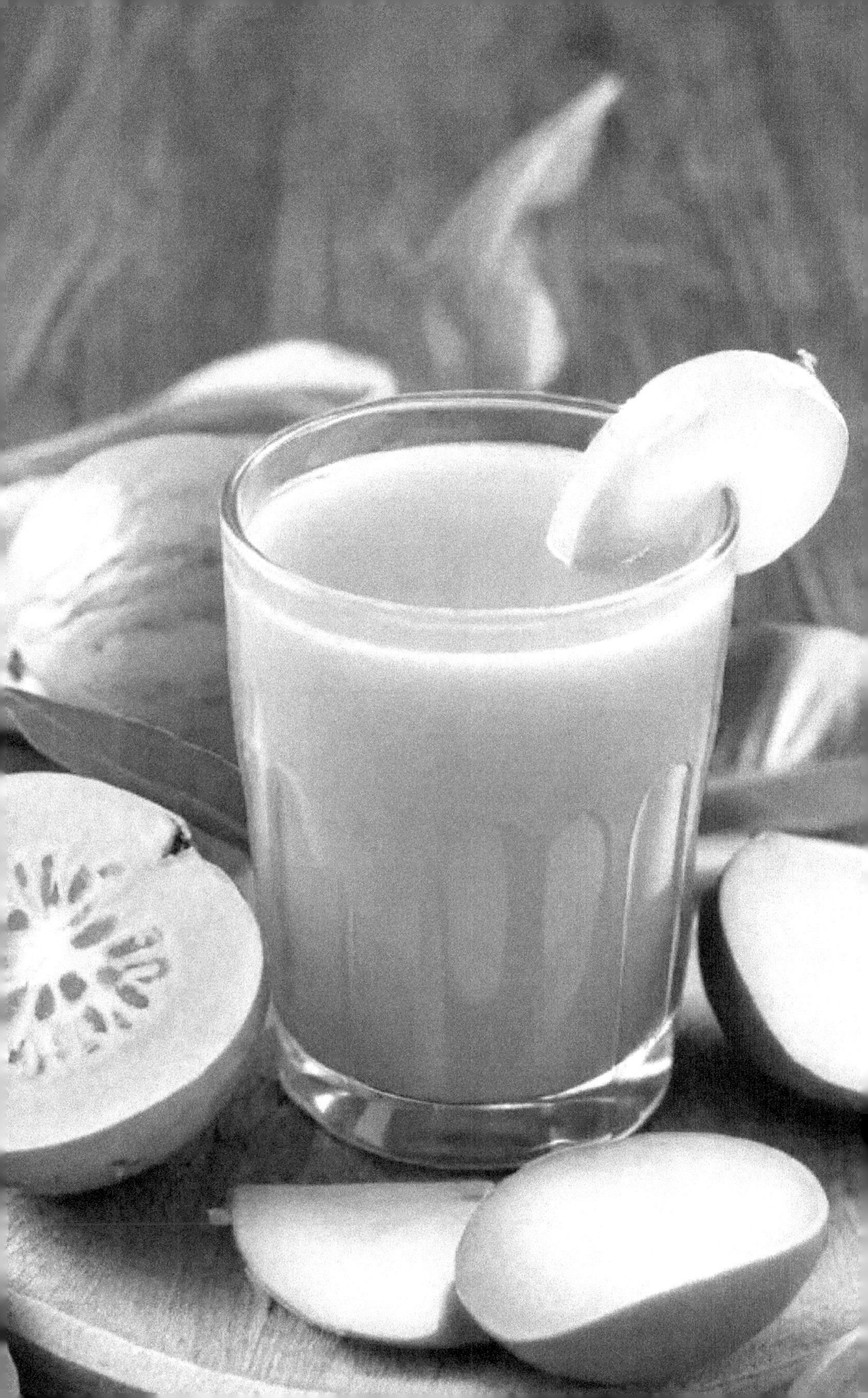

Calming Carrot Apple Juice

This simple juice combines the natural sweetness of carrots with the soothing properties of apple to create a refreshing drink that helps manage acid reflux.

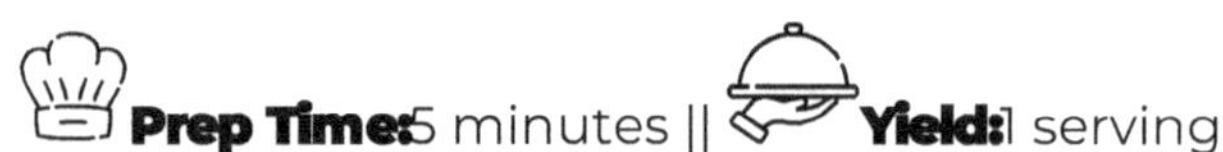
Prep Time: 5 minutes || **Yield:** 1 serving

INGREDIENTS
- 3 large carrots, peeled and chopped
- 1 apple (tart or sweet, depending on preference), cored and chopped
- 1/2 inch knob of ginger, peeled (optional)

INSTRUCTIONS
1. Wash and peel the carrots and apple. Chop them into pieces that will fit comfortably in your juicer.
2. Peel the ginger with a spoon or vegetable peeler, if using.
3. Juice the carrots, apple, and ginger together using a juicer.
4. Enjoy the juice immediately for maximum freshness.

NOTES
- Tart apples, like Granny Smith, can help neutralize stomach acid, while sweeter apples like Fuji can still be tolerated by some. Choose the variety that best suits your taste and acid reflux sensitivity.
- The ginger is optional, but it can provide additional anti-inflammatory benefits. Start with a small piece and add more if desired.
- If you don't have a juicer, you can blend the ingredients with a little water and then strain the pulp. However, juicing provides a more concentrated dose of nutrients.

EXTRA TIPS
- Drink this juice on an empty stomach, at least 30 minutes before a meal, for optimal relief.
- Consider adding a squeeze of lemon for extra flavor, but be mindful that citrus can worsen acid reflux for some people.

Soothing Summer Melon Juice

This light and hydrating juice combines the natural alkalinity of melons with other stomach-friendly ingredients to offer relief from acid reflux symptoms.

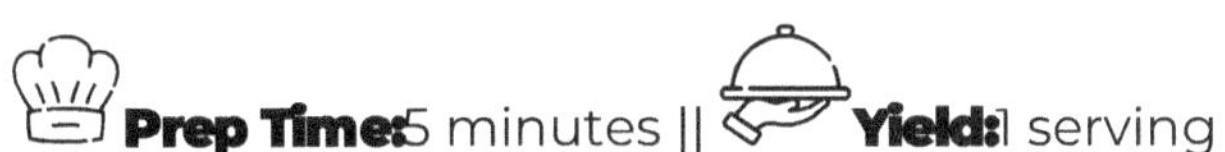
Prep Time: 5 minutes || **Yield:** 1 serving

INGREDIENTS
- 2 cups chopped seedless watermelon
- 1 cup chopped cantaloupe or honeydew melon
- 1/2 cucumber, peeled and chopped (optional)
- 1 sprig of fresh mint (optional)

INSTRUCTIONS
1. Wash and chop the watermelon, cantaloupe/honeydew melon, and cucumber (if using).
2. Wash and add the mint sprig to the juicer, if using.
3. Juice all ingredients together using a juicer.
4. Enjoy the juice immediately for maximum freshness.

NOTES
- Melons are naturally low in acid and high in water content, making them ideal for soothing acid reflux. You can adjust the ratio of watermelon to cantaloupe/honeydew based on your preference.
- The cucumber adds a refreshing twist and additional hydrating benefits, but some people find it slightly irritating for acid reflux. Include it only if tolerated.
- Fresh mint is optional, but it can provide a calming and digestive-aid effect.

EXTRA TIPS
- Drink this juice on an empty stomach, at least 30 minutes before a meal, for optimal relief.
- Consider chilling the ingredients before juicing for an extra refreshing beverage.
- If you don't have a juicer, you can blend the ingredients with a little water and then strain the pulp. However, juicing provides a more concentrated dose of nutrients.

Gentle Aloe Vera Juice

This simple drink utilizes the soothing properties of aloe vera to provide relief from acid reflux discomfort. However, it's important to use aloe vera juice specifically formulated for consumption.

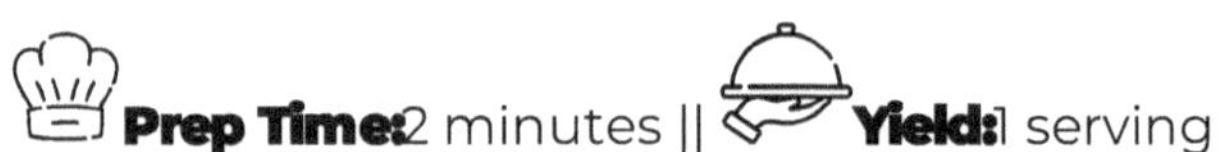

Prep Time: 2 minutes || **Yield:** 1 serving

INGREDIENTS
- 4 ounces 100% pure aloe vera juice (for internal consumption)
- 4 ounces water (or to desired taste)

INSTRUCTIONS
1. **Important:** Purchase aloe vera juice specifically labeled for internal consumption. Do not use juice meant for topical application.
2. Measure out 4 ounces of aloe vera juice.
3. Dilute the juice with 4 ounces of water, or adjust the water content to your taste preference.
4. Enjoy the juice immediately.

NOTES
- Start with a smaller amount of aloe vera juice, like 2 ounces, to assess your tolerance. Some people may experience stomach upset with larger quantities.
- You can adjust the water ratio to dilute the aloe vera juice further if it has a strong flavor.
- Aloe vera juice can interact with certain medications. Consult your doctor before consuming aloe vera juice if you are taking any medications.

EXTRA TIPS
- Drink this juice on an empty stomach, at least 30 minutes before a meal, for optimal relief.
- If you experience any discomfort after consuming aloe vera juice, discontinue use and consult your doctor.

Cabbage Ginger Juice

This invigorating juice combines the potential stomach-soothing properties of cabbage with the anti-inflammatory benefits of ginger to create a flavourful drink that may help manage acid reflux symptoms.

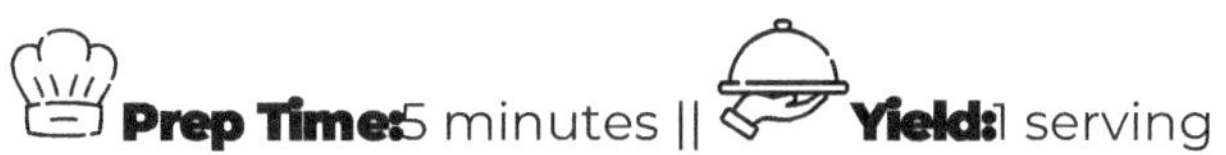

Prep Time: 5 minutes || **Yield:** 1 serving

INGREDIENTS
- 2 large cabbage leaves, washed and roughly chopped
- 1 inch knob of ginger, peeled and chopped

INSTRUCTIONS
1. Wash the cabbage leaves thoroughly and chop them into pieces that will fit comfortably in your juicer.
2. Peel the ginger with a spoon or vegetable peeler.
3. Juice the cabbage leaves and ginger together using a juicer.
4. Enjoy the juice immediately for maximum freshness.

NOTES
- While research on the effectiveness of cabbage juice for acid reflux is limited, some people find it helpful.
- The strong flavor of cabbage can be quite pungent. The ginger helps balance the taste and adds a warming quality. You can adjust the amount of ginger depending on your preference.
- If you don't have a juicer, you can blend the ingredients with a little water and then strain the pulp. However, juicing provides a more concentrated dose of nutrients.

EXTRA TIPS
- Drink this juice on an empty stomach, at least 30 minutes before a meal, for optimal relief.
- Cabbage juice can be slightly high in sugar content. If you have concerns about sugar intake, discuss this with your doctor.
- Start with a smaller amount of cabbage juice, like 4 ounces, to assess your tolerance. Some people may experience bloating or gas.

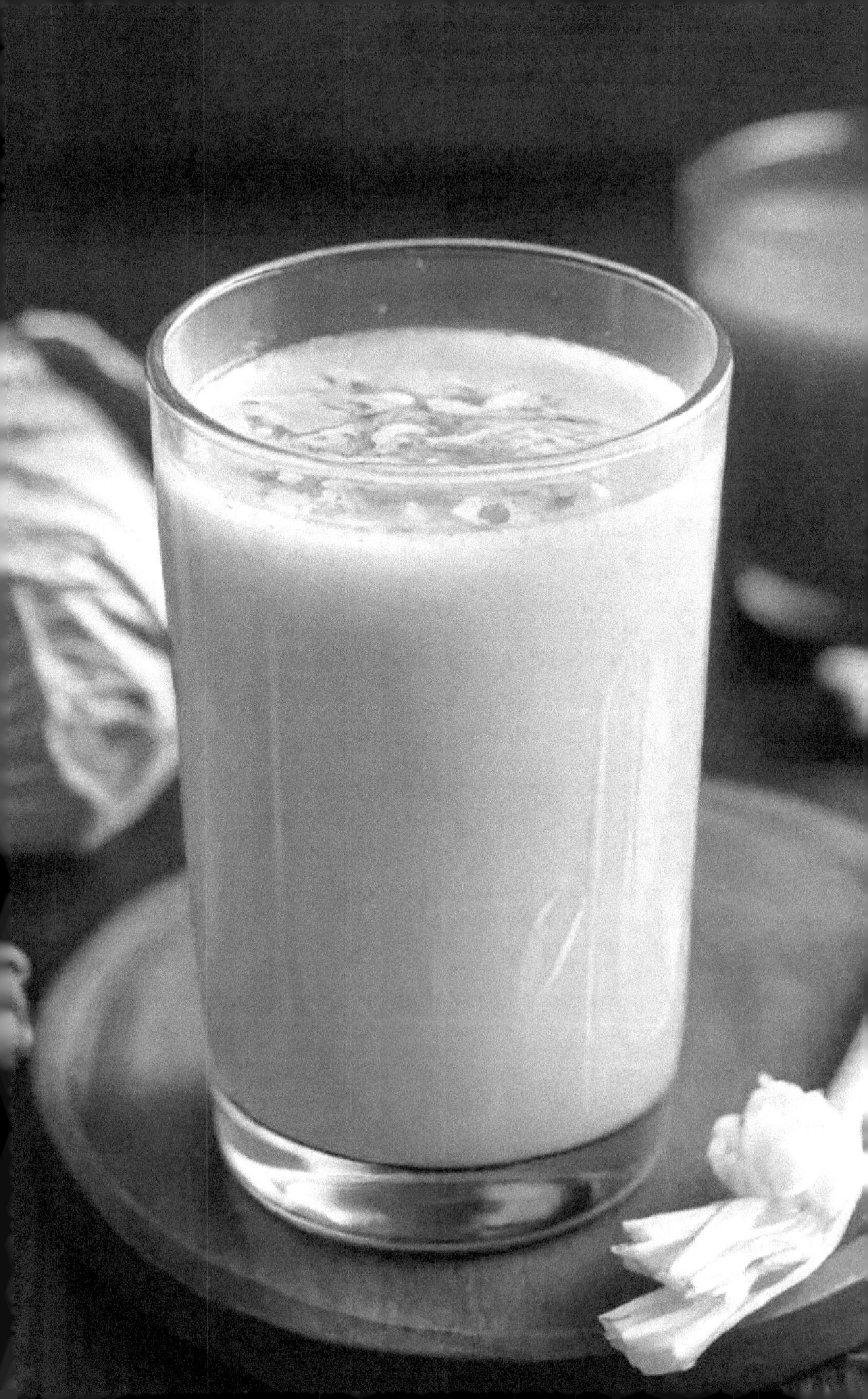

Cooling Cucumber Mint Juice

This refreshing drink harnesses the hydrating and potentially soothing properties of cucumber to help manage acid reflux discomfort.

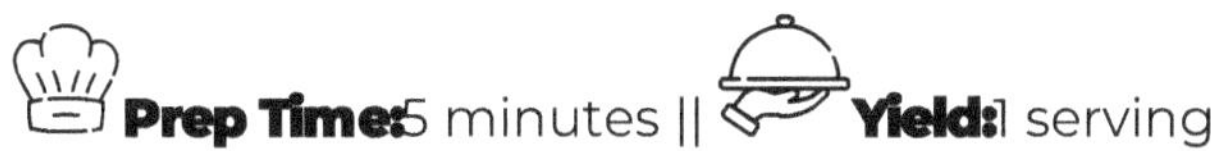

Prep Time: 5 minutes || **Yield:** 1 serving

INGREDIENTS
- 1 large cucumber, peeled and chopped
- 1/2 lemon, juiced (optional)
- Sprig of fresh mint (optional)

INSTRUCTIONS
1. Wash and peel the cucumber. Chop it into pieces that will fit comfortably in your juicer.
2. **Optional:** - Squeeze the juice from half a lemon. Consider omitting the lemon if citrus irritates your acid reflux.
3. Wash and add the mint sprig to the juicer, if using.
4. Juice the cucumber, lemon juice (if using), and mint together using a juicer.
5. Enjoy the juice immediately for maximum freshness.

NOTES
- Cucumbers are naturally high in water content and low in acid, making them a potentially helpful beverage for acid reflux.
- The lemon juice adds a touch of flavor, but it is acidic. If citrus irritates your acid reflux, omit it entirely.
- Fresh mint is optional, but it can provide a refreshing taste and potentially aid digestion.

EXTRA TIPS
- Drink this juice on an empty stomach, at least 30 minutes before a meal, for optimal relief.
- Consider chilling the cucumber before juicing for an extra refreshing beverage.
- If you don't have a juicer, you can blend the ingredients with a little water and then strain the pulp. However, juicing provides a more concentrated dose of nutrients.

Earthy Beet Ginger Juice

This vibrant juice combines the potential benefits of beets for overall gut health with the anti-inflammatory properties of ginger to create a flavourful drink that may help manage acid reflux symptoms.

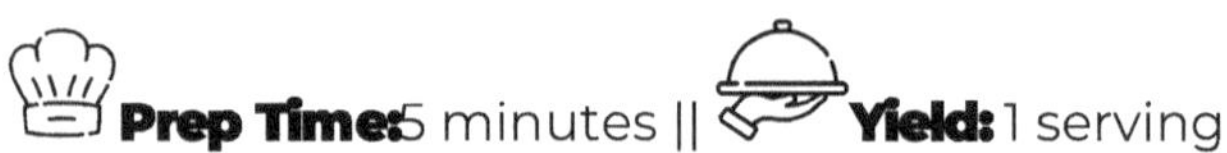
Prep Time: 5 minutes || **Yield:** 1 serving

INGREDIENTS
- 1 medium beet, peeled and chopped
- 1 inch knob of ginger, peeled and chopped
- 1 apple (tart or sweet, depending on preference), cored and chopped (optional)

INSTRUCTIONS
1. Wash, peel, and chop the beet and ginger into pieces that will fit comfortably in your juicer.
2. Core and chop the apple (optional). Choose a tart apple variety like Granny Smith for a potentially acid-neutralizing effect, or a sweeter variety like Fuji if tolerated.
3. Juice the beet, ginger, and apple (if using) together using a juicer.
4. Enjoy the juice immediately for maximum freshness.

NOTES
- While research on the direct impact of beet juice on acid reflux is limited, some people find it beneficial for gut health, which can indirectly influence acid reflux.
- Beets can have an earthy flavor. The ginger helps balance the taste and adds a warming quality. You can adjust the amount of ginger depending on your preference.
- The apple (optional) adds sweetness and additional nutrients. However, some may find apples trigger their acid reflux. Choose a tart variety or omit it entirely if needed.

EXTRA TIPS
- Drink this juice on an empty stomach, at least 30 minutes before a meal, for optimal relief.
- Start with a smaller amount of beet juice, like 4 ounces, to assess your tolerance. Some people may experience bloating or discoloration in their urine due to beet pigments (which is harmless).

Sweet and Soothing Pear Juice

This gentle juice leverages the naturally low-acid properties of pears to offer a calming beverage that may help manage acid reflux discomfort.

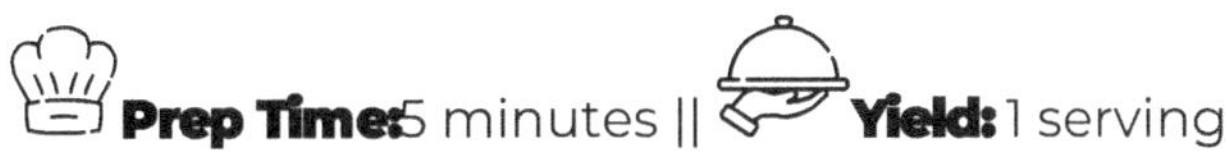

Prep Time: 5 minutes || **Yield:** 1 serving

INGREDIENTS
- 2 ripe pears, peeled and cored

INSTRUCTIONS
1. Wash, peel, and core the pears. Cut them into pieces that will fit comfortably in your juicer.
2. Juice the pears using a juicer.
3. Enjoy the juice immediately for maximum freshness.

NOTES
- Pears are a great choice for people with acid reflux because they are naturally low in acid content.
- The juice may not be very sweet on its own. If desired, you can add a squeeze of honey or a splash of apple juice for additional flavor (be mindful if you have severe acid reflux).

EXTRA TIPS
- Drink this juice on an empty stomach, at least 30 minutes before a meal, for optimal relief.
- Consider chilling the pears before juicing for an extra refreshing beverage.
- If you don't have a juicer, you can blend the pears with a little water and then strain the pulp. However, juicing provides a more concentrated dose of nutrients.

Watermelon Cooler

This hydrating juice harnesses the natural alkalinity of watermelon to create a delicious and potentially soothing beverage for managing acid reflux discomfort.

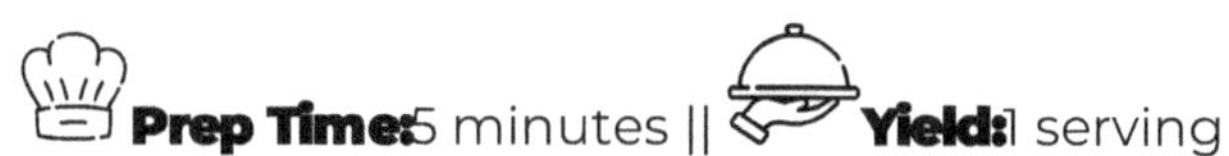

Prep Time: 5 minutes || **Yield:** 1 serving

INGREDIENTS
- 2 cups chopped seedless watermelon
- 1 sprig of fresh mint (optional)

INSTRUCTIONS
1. Wash and chop the watermelon into pieces that will fit comfortably in your juicer.
2. Wash and add the mint sprig to the juicer, if using.
3. Juice the watermelon and mint together using a juicer.
4. Enjoy the juice immediately for maximum freshness.

NOTES
- Watermelon is a superstar for acid reflux sufferers! It's naturally low in acid and high in water content, which can help dilute stomach acid and soothe irritation.
- The mint sprig (optional) adds a refreshing touch and may aid digestion.

EXTRA TIPS
- Drink this juice on an empty stomach, at least 30 minutes before a meal, for optimal relief.
- Consider chilling the watermelon before juicing for an extra refreshing beverage.
- If you don't have a juicer, you can blend the watermelon with a little water and then strain the pulp. However, juicing provides a more concentrated dose of nutrients.

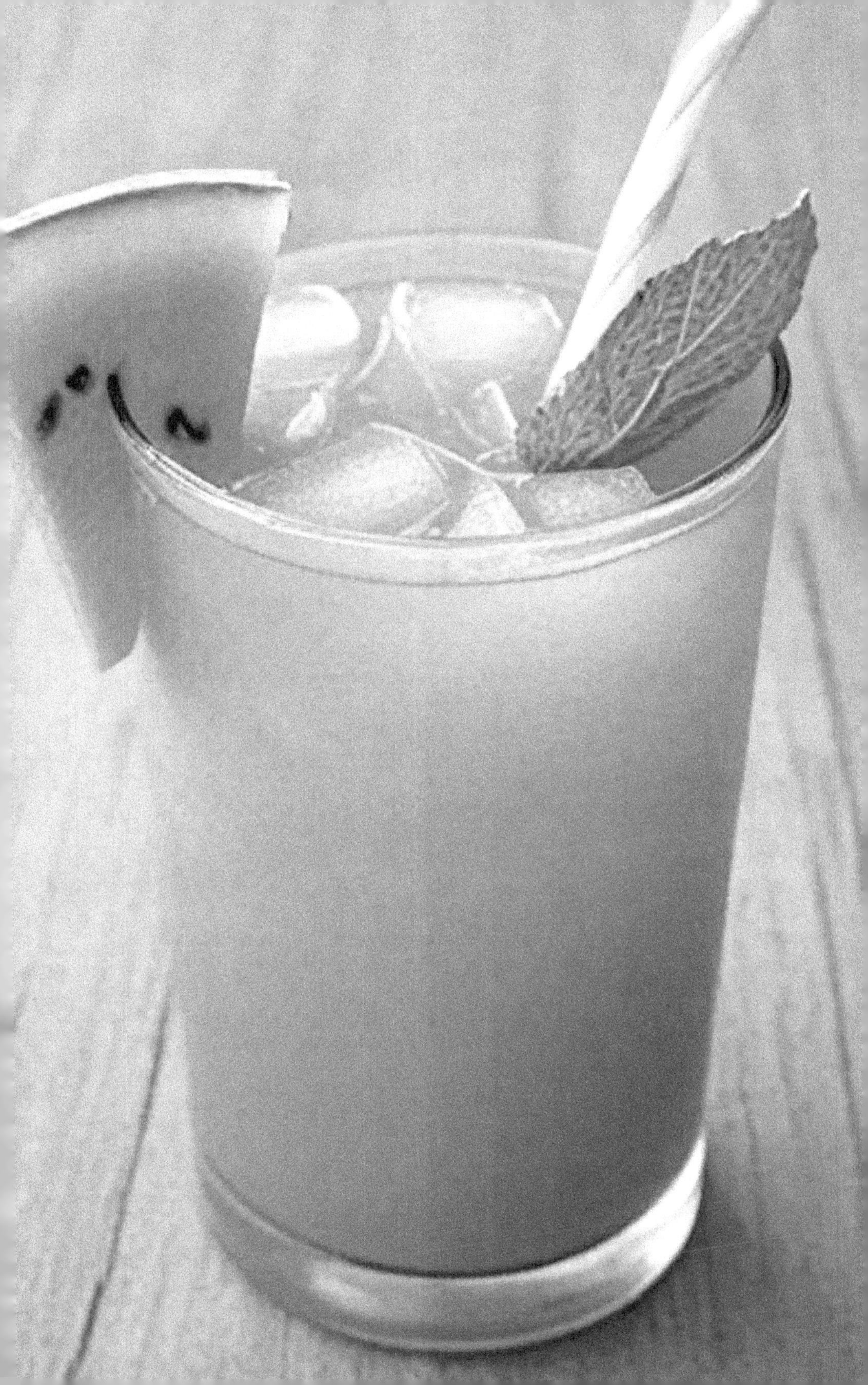

Calming Celery Juice

This simple juice leverages the potential benefits of celery to create a refreshing and potentially helpful beverage for managing acid reflux symptoms.

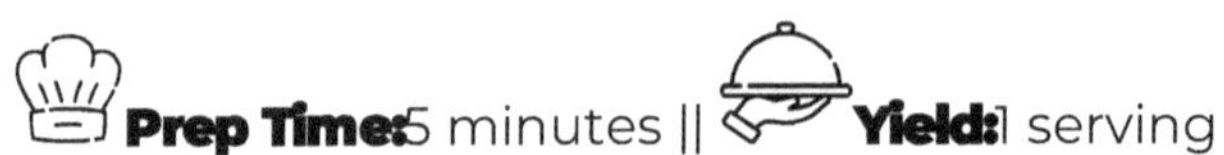

Prep Time: 5 minutes || **Yield:** 1 serving

INGREDIENTS
- 2 large stalks celery, washed and chopped

INSTRUCTIONS
1. Wash and chop the celery stalks into pieces that will fit comfortably in your juicer.
2. Juice the celery using a juicer.
3. Enjoy the juice immediately for maximum freshness.

NOTES
- While research on the direct impact of celery juice on acid reflux is ongoing, some proponents believe it may help by:
   - **Hydrating:** Celery's high water content can help dilute stomach acid and soothe irritation.
   - **Alkaline Properties:** Some sources suggest celery has an alkalizing effect in the body, potentially helping to neutralize stomach acid.

EXTRA TIPS
- Drink this juice on an empty stomach, at least 30 minutes before a meal, for optimal relief.
- Celery juice can have a strong flavor. You can dilute it with a splash of water or add a squeeze of lemon or lime juice (be mindful of citrus if it irritates your reflux).
- Celery juice may interact with certain medications, particularly blood thinners. Consult your doctor before consuming celery juice if you are taking any medications.

Sweet and Soothing Mango Juice

This tropical drink utilizes the potential benefits of ripe mangoes to create a delicious and potentially acid-reflux-friendly juice.

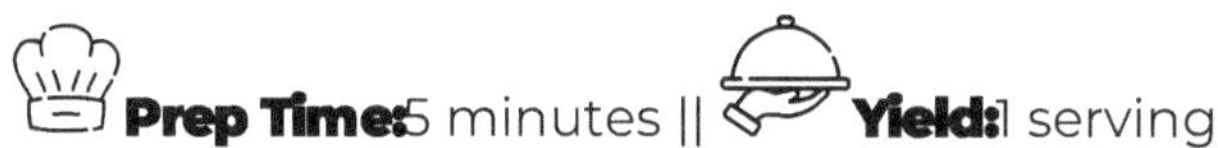

INGREDIENTS
- 1 ripe mango, peeled and pitted

INSTRUCTIONS
1. Wash, peel, and pit the mango. Cut it into pieces that will fit comfortably in your juicer.
2. Juice the mango using a juicer.
3. Enjoy the juice immediately for maximum freshness.

NOTES
- Unlike citrus fruits, ripe mangoes are generally well-tolerated by individuals with acid reflux. This is because they have a relatively low acidity level, typically falling between 5.4 and 6.7 on the pH scale (considered low to moderately acidic).
- The sweetness of ripe mangoes can be a delightful alternative to more tart fruits that may trigger acid reflux.

EXTRA TIPS
- Drink this juice on an empty stomach, at least 30 minutes before a meal, for optimal relief.
- If the mango is not very sweet, consider adding a squeeze of lime juice (be mindful of citrus if it irritates your reflux) or a touch of honey for additional flavor.
- Start with a smaller amount of mango juice, like 4 ounces, to assess your tolerance. Some people may experience digestive issues with large quantities of fruit juice.

Papaya Juice

This vibrant juice harnesses the potential digestive benefits of papaya to create a refreshing and potentially helpful beverage for managing acid reflux symptoms.

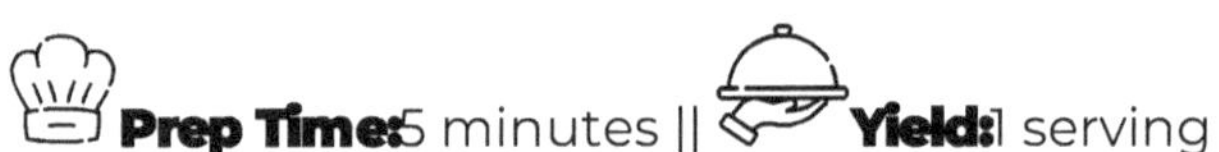

INGREDIENTS
- 1 ripe papaya, peeled and seeded

INSTRUCTIONS
1. Wash, peel, and remove the seeds from the papaya. Cut it into pieces that will fit comfortably in your juicer.
2. Juice the papaya using a juicer.
3. Enjoy the juice immediately for maximum freshness.

NOTES
- Papaya contains papain, an enzyme known to aid digestion. While research on its direct impact on acid reflux is not conclusive, some studies suggest it may help with overall digestive discomfort, potentially alleviating acid reflux symptoms.
- Papaya is also a good source of fiber, which can promote healthy digestion and potentially reduce bloating, a common side effect of acid reflux.

EXTRA TIPS
- Drink this juice on an empty stomach, at least 30 minutes before a meal, for optimal relief.
- Papaya can have a subtle sweetness. If desired, you can add a squeeze of lime juice (be mindful of citrus if it irritates your reflux) for additional flavor.
- Papaya leaves, sometimes used in teas or supplements, are not recommended for acid reflux. Stick to ripe papaya fruit for potential digestive benefits.

Strawberry Juice

This delightful juice leverages the potential benefits of strawberries to create a refreshing and potentially acid-reflux-friendly beverage.

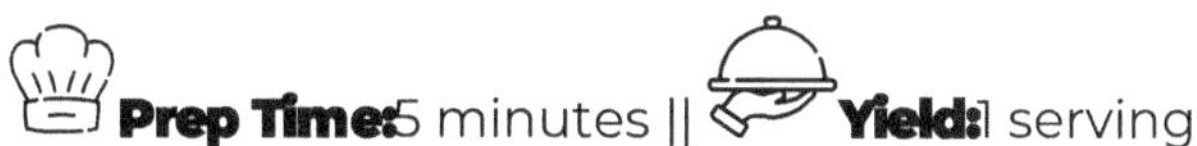

Prep Time: 5 minutes || **Yield:** 1 serving

INGREDIENTS
- 2 cups fresh strawberries, washed and hulled

INSTRUCTIONS
1. Wash the strawberries thoroughly and remove the hulls (green leafy tops).
2. Juice the strawberries using a juicer.
3. Enjoy the juice immediately for maximum freshness.

NOTES
- Strawberries are generally considered a good choice for people with acid reflux. This is because they have a relatively low acidity level, typically falling between 3.5 and 4.5 on the pH scale (considered mildly acidic).
- The natural sweetness of strawberries can be a delightful alternative to more tart fruits that may trigger acid reflux.

EXTRA TIPS
- Drink this juice on an empty stomach, at least 30 minutes before a meal, for optimal relief.
- If the strawberries are not very sweet, consider adding a squeeze of lime juice (be mindful of citrus if it irritates your reflux) or a touch of honey for additional flavor.
- Start with a smaller amount of strawberry juice, like 4 ounces, to assess your tolerance. Some people may experience digestive issues with large quantities of fruit juice.

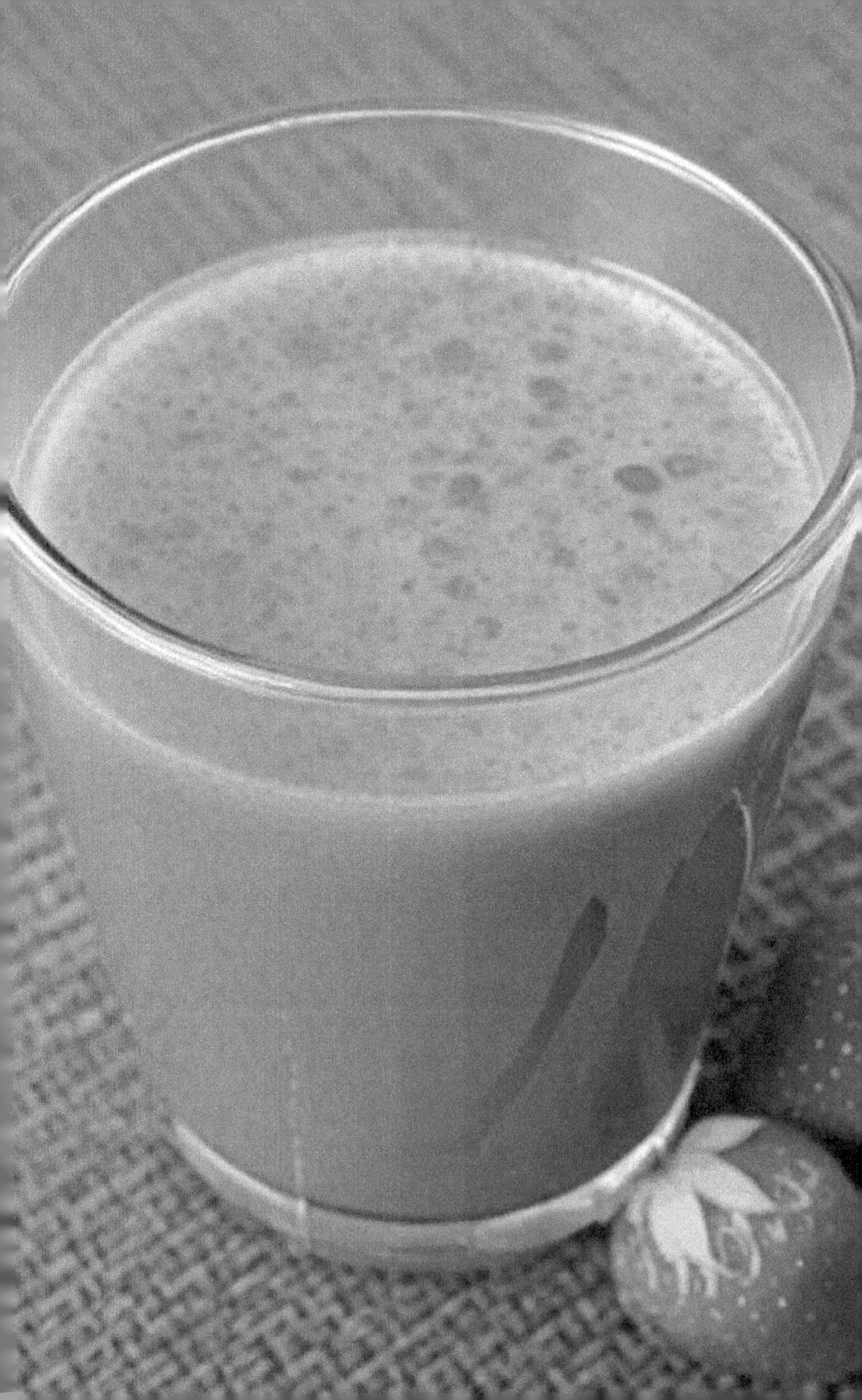

Soothing Green Spinach, Apple, & Cucumber Juice

This nutrient-packed juice utilizes the potential benefits of spinach to create a refreshing and potentially helpful drink for managing acid reflux symptoms.

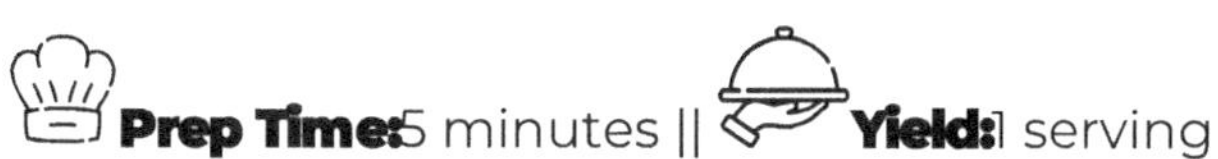

Prep Time: 5 minutes || **Yield:** 1 serving

INGREDIENTS
- 2 cups fresh spinach, washed
- 1 apple (tart or sweet, depending on preference) - optional
- 1/2 cucumber - optional (consider omitting if cucumber irritates your reflux)
- Splash of water (optional)

INSTRUCTIONS
1. Wash the spinach thoroughly.
2. Core and chop the apple (optional). Choose a tart apple variety like Granny Smith for a potentially acid-neutralizing effect, or a sweeter variety like Fuji if tolerated.
3. Peel and chop the cucumber (optional), omitting it if it irritates your reflux.
4. Juice the spinach, apple (if using), and cucumber (if using) together using a juicer. You may need to add a splash of water to aid juicing.
5. Enjoy the juice immediately for maximum freshness.

NOTES
- Spinach is a good source of vitamins and minerals, and some studies suggest it may help with digestion. However, research on its direct impact on acid reflux is limited.
- Juicing removes most of the fiber from spinach, which can be beneficial for some people with acid reflux who struggle with bulky foods. However, fiber can also play a role in digestion, so consider including whole spinach in your diet alongside the juice.
- The apple (optional) adds sweetness and additional nutrients. However, some may find apples trigger their acid reflux. Choose a tart variety or omit it entirely if needed.

EXTRA TIPS

- Drink this juice on an empty stomach, at least 30 minutes before a meal, for optimal relief.
- Start with a smaller amount of spinach juice, like 4 ounces, to assess your tolerance. Some people may experience bloating or gas from concentrated green juices.
- Consider adding a pinch of ginger to the juice for a warming and potentially anti-inflammatory effect.
- Spinach is high in vitamin K, which can interfere with blood thinners. Consult your doctor before consuming spinach juice if you are taking blood thinners.

Green Juice III

This hydrating juice combines the potential benefits of several ingredients to create a delicious and potentially acid-reflux-friendly beverage.

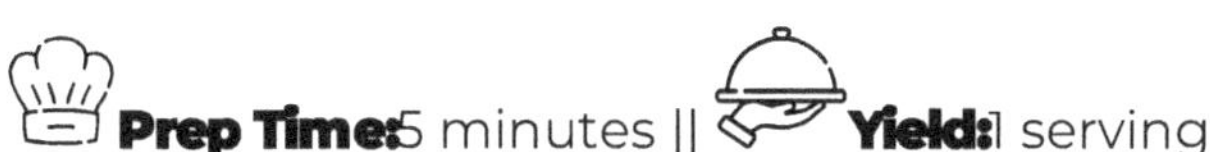

Prep Time: 5 minutes || **Yield:** 1 serving

INGREDIENTS
- 1 large cucumber, peeled and chopped
- 2 stalks celery, washed and chopped
- 1 cup fresh spinach, washed
- 1 pear, peeled and cored

INSTRUCTIONS
1. Wash and chop the cucumber, celery, and spinach.
2. Peel, core, and chop the pear.
3. Juice all ingredients together using a juicer.
4. Enjoy the juice immediately for maximum freshness.

NOTES
- **Cucumber:** Naturally low in acid and high in water content, cucumber helps dilute stomach acid and soothe irritation.
- **Celery:** High water content and potentially has alkaline properties, which may help neutralize stomach acid.
- **Spinach:** While research is limited, some studies suggest spinach may aid digestion, potentially relieving acid reflux discomfort.
- **Pear:** A low-acid fruit that provides natural sweetness without triggering reflux in most people.

EXTRA TIPS
- Drink this juice on an empty stomach, at least 30 minutes before a meal, for optimal relief.
- Start with a smaller amount of juice, like 8 ounces, to assess your tolerance, especially for the spinach content.
- Consider chilling the ingredients before juicing for an extra refreshing beverage.

IMPORTANT: - Spinach is high in vitamin K, which can interfere with blood thinners. Consult your doctor before consuming spinach juice if you are taking blood thinners.

Soothing Green Juice IV

This energizing juice combines the potential benefits of various ingredients to create a flavorful drink that may help manage acid reflux symptoms.

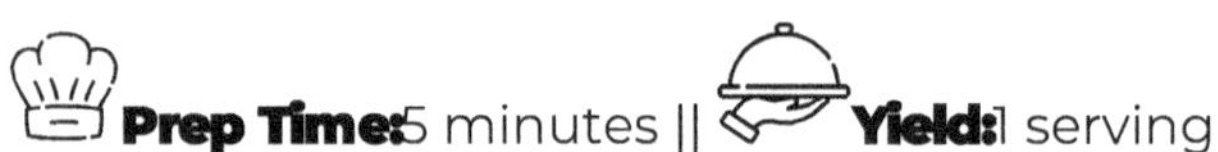

Prep Time: 5 minutes || **Yield:** 1 serving

INGREDIENTS
- 1 cup chopped kale, washed and ribs removed (optional)
- 1 large cucumber, peeled and chopped
- 1 inch knob of ginger, peeled and chopped
- 1 apple (tart or sweet, depending on preference)

INSTRUCTIONS
1. Wash and remove the tough ribs from the kale (optional). You can use a vegetable peeler or simply tear the leaves off the central stem.
2. Core and chop the apple. Choose a tart apple variety like Granny Smith for a potentially acid-neutralizing effect, or a sweeter variety like Fuji if tolerated.
3. Peel and chop the ginger.
4. Juice all ingredients together using a juicer.
5. Enjoy the juice immediately for maximum freshness.

NOTES
- **Kale (optional):** While a powerhouse of nutrients, kale can be high in fiber and irritate some people with acid reflux. Consider omitting it or starting with a very small amount.
- **Cucumber:** Naturally low in acid and high in water content, cucumber helps dilute stomach acid and soothe irritation.
- **Ginger:** Anti-inflammatory properties may help reduce reflux discomfort.
- **Apple:** Choose a tart variety like Granny Smith, which may help neutralize stomach acid. Sweeter apples may trigger reflux in some people.

EXTRA TIPS
- Drink this juice on an empty stomach, at least 30 minutes before a meal, for optimal relief.

- Start with a smaller amount of juice, especially if including kale, to assess your tolerance.
- Consider adding a pinch of turmeric to the juice for additional anti-inflammatory benefits.

IMPORTANT: - Consult your doctor before consuming kale juice if you have any underlying health conditions or are taking medications, particularly blood thinners.

Spinach, Celery, Watermelon & Parsley Juice

This refreshing juice combines the potential benefits of several ingredients to create a hydrating and potentially acid-reflux-friendly beverage.

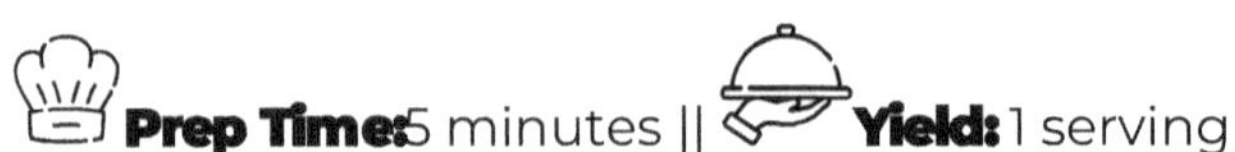

Prep Time: 5 minutes || **Yield:** 1 serving

INGREDIENTS
- 1 cup chopped fresh spinach, washed
- 2 stalks celery, washed and chopped
- 1/4 cup fresh parsley, washed and chopped
- 2 cups chopped seedless watermelon

INSTRUCTIONS
1. Wash all ingredients thoroughly. Chop the spinach, celery, and parsley.
2. Chop the watermelon into pieces that will fit comfortably in your juicer.
3. Juice all ingredients together using a juicer.
4. Enjoy the juice immediately for maximum freshness.

NOTES
- **Spinach:** While research on its direct impact on acid reflux is limited, some studies suggest spinach may aid digestion, potentially relieving acid reflux discomfort.   Note: - Juicing removes most fiber from spinach, so consider including whole spinach in your diet alongside the juice.
- **Celery:** High water content and potentially has alkaline properties, which may help neutralize stomach acid.
- **Parsley:** Traditionally used as a digestive aid, parsley may offer some relief from bloating and discomfort associated with acid reflux.
- **Watermelon:** Naturally low in acid and high in water content, watermelon helps dilute stomach acid and soothe irritation.

EXTRA TIPS
- Drink this juice on an empty stomach, at least 30 minutes before a meal, for optimal relief.
- Start with a smaller amount of juice, especially if including spinach, to assess your tolerance.
- Spinach is high in vitamin K, which can interfere with blood thinners. Consult your doctor before consuming spinach juice if you are taking blood thinners.

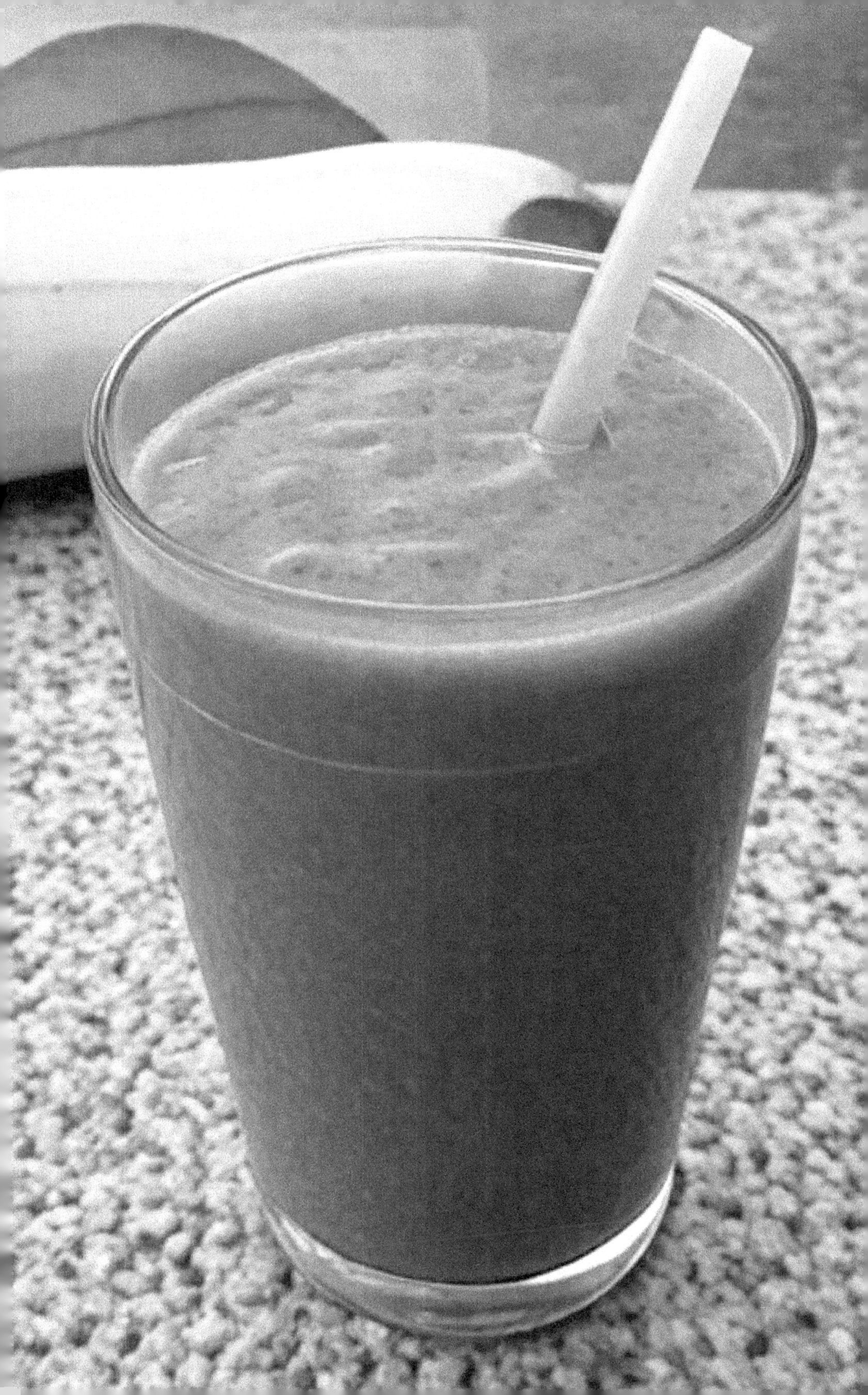

Autumnal Juice

This vibrant juice combines the potential benefits of several ingredients to create a flavourful and potentially acid-reflux-friendly beverage.

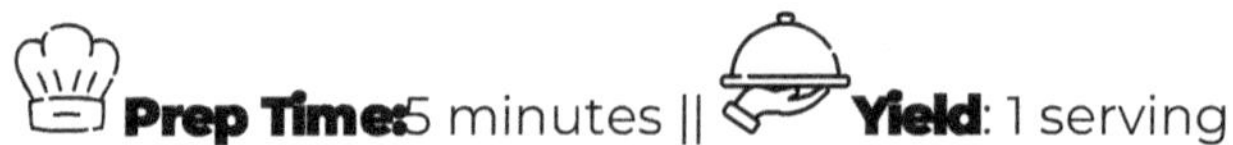
Prep Time: 5 minutes || **Yield**: 1 serving

INGREDIENTS
- 2 large carrots, peeled and chopped
- 1 medium sweet potato, peeled and chopped
- 1 apple (tart or sweet, depending on preference)
- 1 inch knob of turmeric, peeled and chopped (optional)

INSTRUCTIONS
1. Wash, peel, and chop the carrots and sweet potato.
2. Core and chop the apple. Choose a tart apple variety like Granny Smith for a potentially acid-neutralizing effect, or a sweeter variety like Fuji if tolerated.
3. Peel and chop the turmeric (optional).
4. Juice all ingredients together using a juicer.
5. Enjoy the juice immediately for maximum freshness.

NOTES
- **Carrots:** Naturally high in beta-carotene and have a low acidity level, potentially aiding digestion without triggering reflux.
- **Sweet Potato:** Similar to carrots, sweet potatoes are low-acid and a good source of vitamins and minerals.
- **Apple:** Choose a tart variety like Granny Smith, which may help neutralize stomach acid. Sweeter apples may trigger reflux in some people.
- **Turmeric (optional):** Known for its anti-inflammatory properties, turmeric may help reduce reflux discomfort. However, high doses can irritate the stomach in some individuals.

EXTRA TIPS
- Drink this juice on an empty stomach, at least 30 minutes before a meal, for optimal relief.
- Start with a smaller amount of juice, especially if including turmeric, to assess your tolerance.

- Consider adding a squeeze of ginger for an extra anti-inflammatory boost.
- Consult your doctor before consuming turmeric juice if you have any underlying health conditions or are taking medications, particularly blood thinners.

Mint, Cucumber & Green Apple Juice

This invigorating juice combines the potential benefits of three ingredients to create a delicious and potentially acid-reflux-friendly beverage.

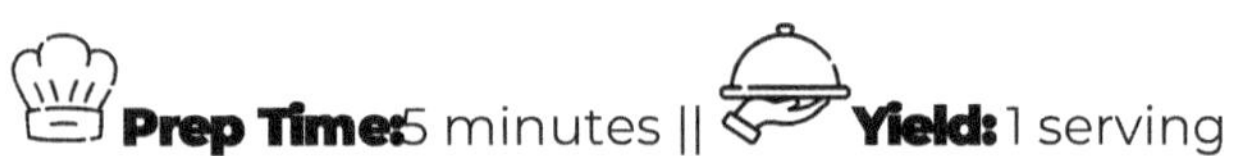
Prep Time: 5 minutes || **Yield:** 1 serving

INGREDIENTS
- 1 large cucumber, peeled and chopped
- 1 green apple, cored and chopped (tart variety recommended)
- Sprig of fresh mint (optional)

INSTRUCTIONS
1. Wash and peel the cucumber. Chop it into pieces that will fit comfortably in your juicer.
2. Core and chop the green apple. Choose a tart variety like Granny Smith, which may help neutralize stomach acid.
3. Wash and add the mint sprig to the juicer, if using.
4. Juice all ingredients together using a juicer.
5. Enjoy the juice immediately for maximum freshness.

NOTES
- **Cucumber:** Naturally low in acid and high in water content, cucumber helps dilute stomach acid and soothe irritation.
- **Green Apple (tart):** Tart green apples are lower in acid than sweeter varieties and may help neutralize stomach acid.
- **Mint (optional):** While research is limited, some people find mint aids digestion and provides a refreshing taste.

EXTRA TIPS
- Drink this juice on an empty stomach, at least 30 minutes before a meal, for optimal relief.
- Start with a smaller amount of juice, especially if including mint, to assess your tolerance. Mint can be strong for some people.
- Consider chilling the ingredients before juicing for an extra refreshing beverage.

IMPORTANT: Peppermint may relax the lower esophageal sphincter (LES) in some people, worsening reflux symptoms. If you experience any discomfort after consuming mint, discontinue use.

Aloe, Cucumber, Ginger & Melon Juice

This intriguing juice combines the potential benefits of aloe vera, cucumber, ginger, and melon to create a flavorful drink that may offer some relief from acid reflux symptoms.

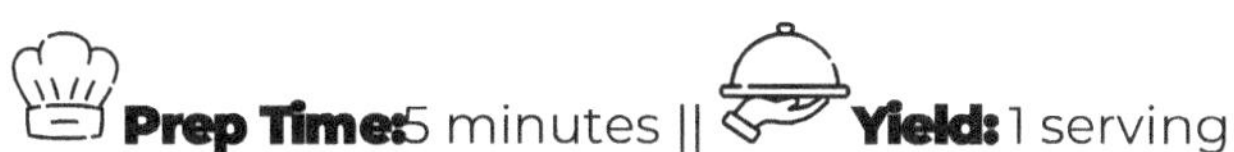

Prep Time: 5 minutes || **Yield:** 1 serving

INGREDIENTS
- 2 large aloe vera leaves (for internal consumption, peeled) OR - 4 ounces 100% pure aloe vera juice (for internal consumption)
- 1 large cucumber, peeled and chopped
- 1 inch knob of ginger, peeled and chopped
- 2 cups chopped seedless watermelon (or cantaloupe, honeydew)

INSTRUCTIONS
Important Note: Use only aloe vera designated for internal consumption. Do not use aloe vera gel meant for topical application.

Option 1: Using Aloe Vera Leaves
1. Wash the aloe vera leaves thoroughly. Using a sharp knife, carefully peel away the tough outer rind, leaving behind the clear inner gel.
2. Chop the aloe vera gel into pieces that will fit comfortably in your juicer.

Option 2: Using Aloe Vera Juice
Skip steps 1 & 2 and simply measure out 4 ounces of 100% pure aloe vera juice (for internal consumption).
3. Wash, peel, and chop the cucumber and ginger.
4. Chop the watermelon (or cantaloupe, honeydew) into pieces that will fit comfortably in your juicer.
5. Juice all ingredients together using a juicer.
6. Enjoy the juice immediately for maximum freshness.

NOTES
- **Aloe Vera (use with caution**): While some studies suggest aloe vera may help with heartburn, research is ongoing. It's important to use aloe vera specifically processed for internal consumption to avoid adverse effects.
- **Cucumber:** Naturally low in acid and high in water content, cucumber helps dilute stomach acid and soothe irritation.

- Ginger: Known for its anti-inflammatory properties, ginger may help reduce reflux discomfort.

- Melon (Watermelon, Cantaloupe, Honeydew): All three melons are naturally low in acid and high in water content, potentially aiding digestion without triggering reflux.

EXTRA TIPS

- Drink this juice on an empty stomach, at least 30 minutes before a meal, for optimal relief.
- Start with a smaller amount of juice, especially if including aloe vera, to assess your tolerance. Aloe vera can have laxative effects in some people.
- Consider chilling the ingredients before juicing for an extra refreshing beverage.
- Aloe vera can interact with certain medications. Consult your doctor before consuming aloe vera juice if you are taking any medications.
- Pregnant or breastfeeding women should avoid aloe vera juice.

Cooling Green Juice V

This hydrating juice combines the potential benefits of several ingredients to create a delicious and potentially acid-reflux-friendly beverage.

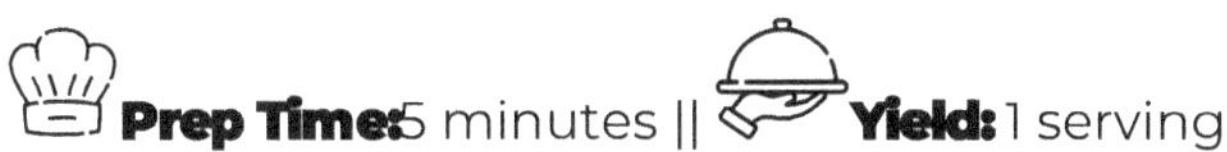 **Prep Time:** 5 minutes || **Yield:** 1 serving

INGREDIENTS
- 1 cup chopped fresh spinach, washed
- 1 large cucumber, peeled and chopped
- 1 medium zucchini, washed and chopped (ends trimmed)
- Sprig of fresh mint (optional)

INSTRUCTIONS
1. Wash all ingredients thoroughly. Chop the spinach, cucumber, and zucchini.
2. Wash and add the mint sprig to the juicer, if using.
3. Juice all ingredients together using a juicer.
4. Enjoy the juice immediately for maximum freshness.

NOTES
- **Spinach:** While research on its direct impact on acid reflux is limited, some studies suggest spinach may aid digestion, potentially relieving acid reflux discomfort.   Note: - Juicing removes most fiber from spinach, so consider including whole spinach in your diet alongside the juice.
- **Cucumber:** Naturally low in acid and high in water content, cucumber helps dilute stomach acid and soothe irritation.
- **Zucchini:** Similar to cucumber, zucchini is low in acid and high in water content, offering hydration without triggering reflux in most people.
- **Mint (optional):** While research is limited, some people find mint aids digestion and provides a refreshing taste.

EXTRA TIPS
- Drink this juice on an empty stomach, at least 30 minutes before a meal, for optimal relief.
- Start with a smaller amount of juice, especially if including spinach, to assess your tolerance.

- Consider chilling the ingredients before juicing for an extra refreshing beverage.
- Spinach is high in vitamin K, which can interfere with blood thinners. Consult your doctor before consuming spinach juice if you are taking blood thinners.

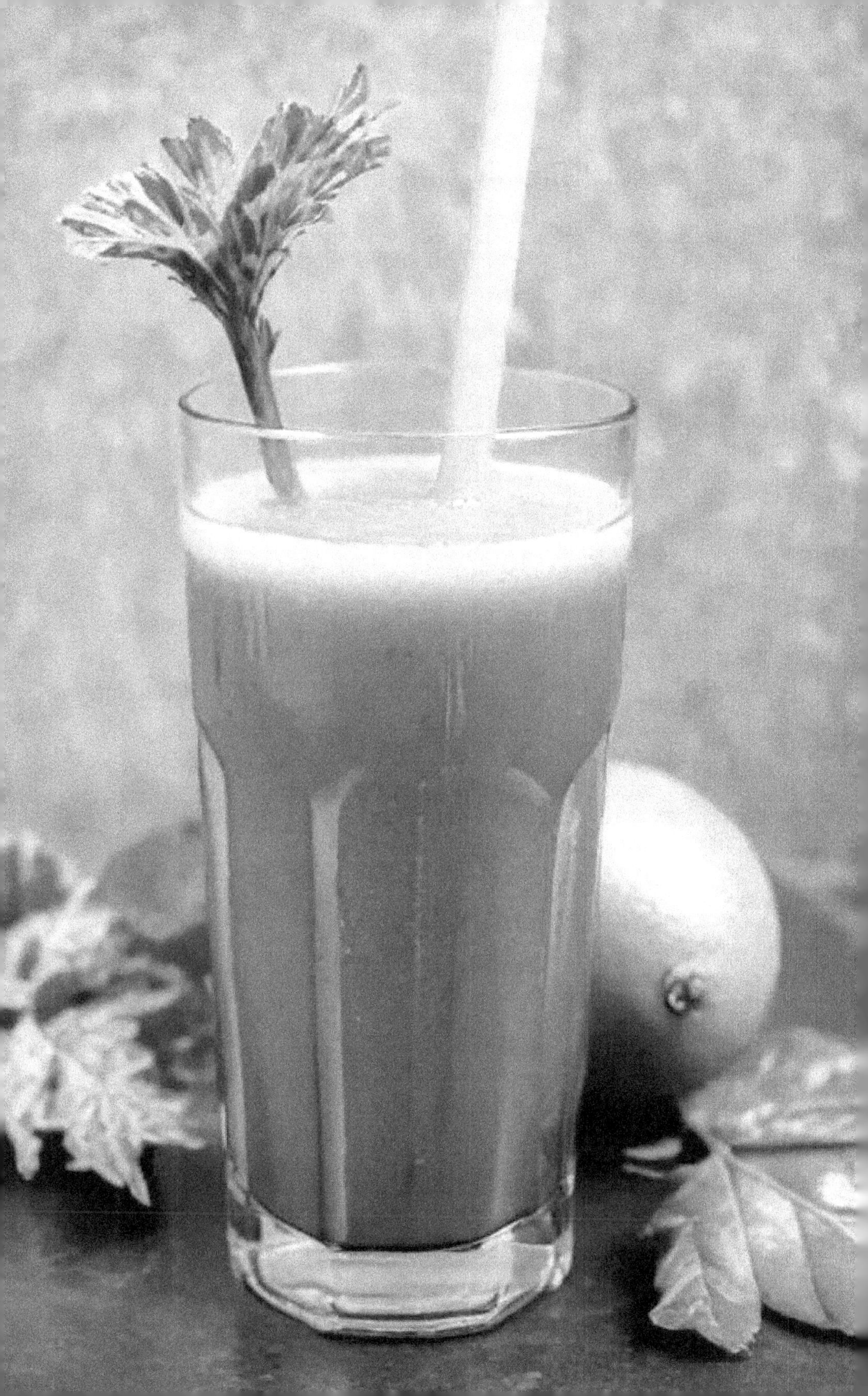

Watermelon, Ginger & Basil Juice

This delightful juice combines the potential benefits of several ingredients to create a delicious and potentially acid-reflux-friendly beverage.

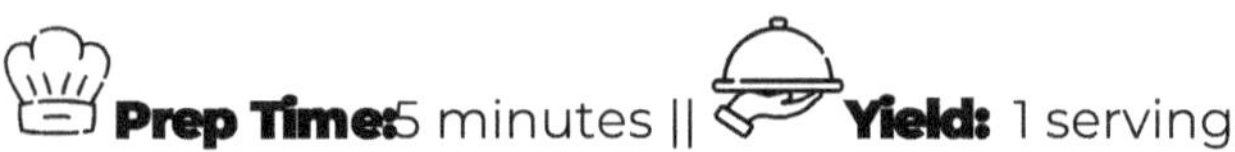

Prep Time: 5 minutes || **Yield:** 1 serving

INGREDIENTS
- 2 cups chopped seedless watermelon
- 1 large cucumber, peeled and chopped
- 1 inch knob of ginger, peeled and chopped
- 1/4 cup fresh basil leaves, washed

INSTRUCTIONS
1. Wash and chop the watermelon, cucumber, and ginger.
2. Wash the basil leaves.
3. Juice all ingredients together using a juicer.
4. Enjoy the juice immediately for maximum freshness.

NOTES
- **Watermelon:** Naturally low in acid and high in water content, watermelon helps dilute stomach acid and soothe irritation.
- **Cucumber:** Naturally low in acid and high in water content, cucumber helps dilute stomach acid and soothe irritation.
- **Ginger:** Known for its anti-inflammatory properties, ginger may help reduce reflux discomfort.
- **Basil:** While research is limited, some find basil soothing for digestion and adds a refreshing flavor.

EXTRA TIPS
- Drink this juice on an empty stomach, at least 30 minutes before a meal, for optimal relief.
- Start with a smaller amount of juice, especially if including ginger, to assess your tolerance. Ginger can be strong for some people.
- Consider chilling the ingredients before juicing for an extra refreshing beverage.

Pear, Cucumber, Fennel & Mint Juice

This delightful juice combines the potential benefits of several ingredients to create a delicious and potentially acid-reflux-friendly beverage.

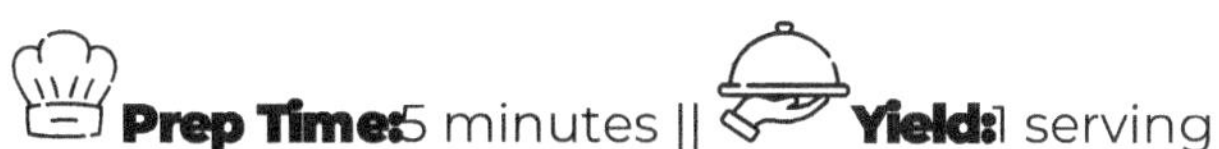

Prep Time: 5 minutes || **Yield:** 1 serving

INGREDIENTS
- 1 ripe pear, peeled and cored
- 1 large cucumber, peeled and chopped
- 1/2 bulb fennel, trimmed and chopped
- Sprig of fresh mint (optional)

INSTRUCTIONS
1. Wash and chop the cucumber and fennel. Peel, core, and chop the pear.
2. Wash and add the mint sprig to the juicer, if using.
3. Juice all ingredients together using a juicer.
4. Enjoy the juice immediately for maximum freshness.

NOTES
- **Pear:** - Naturally low in acid and a good source of fiber, pear adds sweetness without triggering reflux in most people.
- **Cucumber:** - Naturally low in acid and high in water content, cucumber helps dilute stomach acid and soothe irritation.
- **Fennel:** - Contains properties that may aid digestion and reduce bloating, a common reflux symptom.
- **Mint (optional):** - While research is limited, some people find mint aids digestion and provides a refreshing taste.

EXTRA TIPS
- Drink this juice on an empty stomach, at least 30 minutes before a meal, for optimal relief.
- Start with a smaller amount of juice, especially if including fennel or mint, to assess your tolerance. Fennel can have a licorice-like flavour that some may find strong, and mint can relax the oesophageal sphincter in some people, worsening reflux.
- Consider chilling the ingredients before juicing for an extra refreshing beverage.

Pear, Cucumber & Mint Refresher

This refreshing juice combines the potential benefits of three ingredients to create a delicious and potentially acid-reflux-friendly beverage.

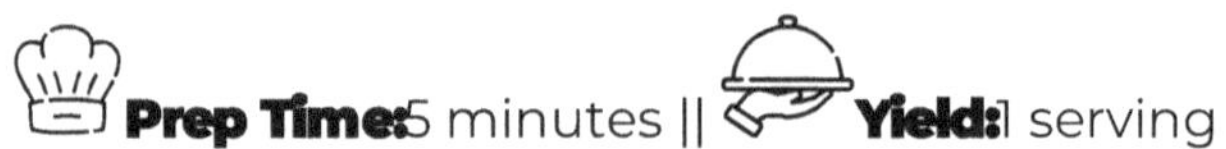

Prep Time: 5 minutes || **Yield:** 1 serving

INGREDIENTS
- 1 ripe pear, peeled and cored
- 1 large cucumber, peeled and chopped
- Sprig of fresh mint (optional)

INSTRUCTIONS
1. Wash and chop the cucumber. Peel, core, and chop the pear.
2. Wash and add the mint sprig to the juicer, if using.
3. Juice all ingredients together using a juicer.
4. Enjoy the juice immediately for maximum freshness.

NOTES
- **Pear:** Naturally low in acid and a good source of fiber, pear adds sweetness without triggering reflux in most people.
- **Cucumber:** Naturally low in acid and high in water content, cucumber helps dilute stomach acid and soothe irritation.
- **Mint (optional):** While research is limited, some people find mint aids digestion and provides a refreshing taste.

EXTRA TIPS
- Drink this juice on an empty stomach, at least 30 minutes before a meal, for optimal relief.
- Start with a smaller amount of juice, especially if including mint, to assess your tolerance. Mint can be strong for some people.
- Consider chilling the ingredients before juicing for an extra refreshing beverage.

Tropical Soother Juice

This drink combines potentially beneficial ingredients for acid reflux relief, but use caution with aloe vera.

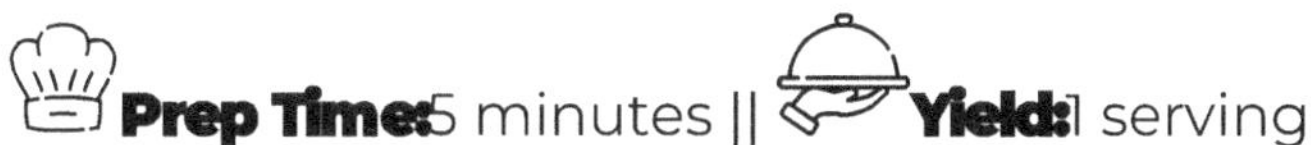

Prep Time: 5 minutes || **Yield:** 1 serving

INGREDIENTS
- Coconut Water (1 cup)
- Cucumber (peeled and chopped, 1 large)
- Aloe Vera (use with caution, see notes below)
    - Option 1: Aloe Vera Leaves (for internal consumption, peeled) - OR -
    - Option 2: 100% Pure Aloe Vera Juice (for internal consumption, 4 ounces)
- Mint (optional, 1 sprig)

INSTRUCTIONS
Important Note: Use only aloe vera designated for internal consumption. Do not use aloe vera gel meant for topical application.

Option 1: Using Aloe Vera Leaves
1. Wash the aloe vera leaves thoroughly. Using a sharp knife, carefully peel away the tough outer rind, leaving behind the clear inner gel.
2. Chop the aloe vera gel into pieces that will fit comfortably in your juicer.

Option 2: Using Aloe Vera Juice
Skip steps 1 & 2 and simply measure out 4 ounces of 100% pure aloe vera juice (for internal consumption).
3. Wash, peel, and chop the cucumber.
4. Wash the mint sprig (optional).
5. Combine all ingredients in a blender and blend until smooth.
   - You may need to add a little extra water for easier blending.

NOTES
- **Coconut Water:** While research is ongoing, some studies suggest coconut water may help with heartburn due to its electrolytes and anti-inflammatory properties.
- **Cucumber:** Naturally low in acid and high in water content, cucumber helps dilute stomach acid and soothe irritation.

-   **Aloe Vera (Use with Caution):** While some studies suggest aloe vera may help with heartburn, research is limited. It's important to use aloe vera specifically processed for internal consumption to avoid adverse effects.

EXTRA TIPS

- Drink this beverage on an empty stomach, at least 30 minutes before a meal, for optimal relief.
- Start with a smaller amount, especially if including aloe vera, to assess your tolerance. Aloe vera can have laxative effects in some people.
- Consider chilling the ingredients before blending for an extra refreshing drink.

IMPORTANT: - Pregnant or breastfeeding women should avoid aloe vera juice.
- Blending is recommended over juicing for this recipe, as aloe vera gel doesn't juice well.

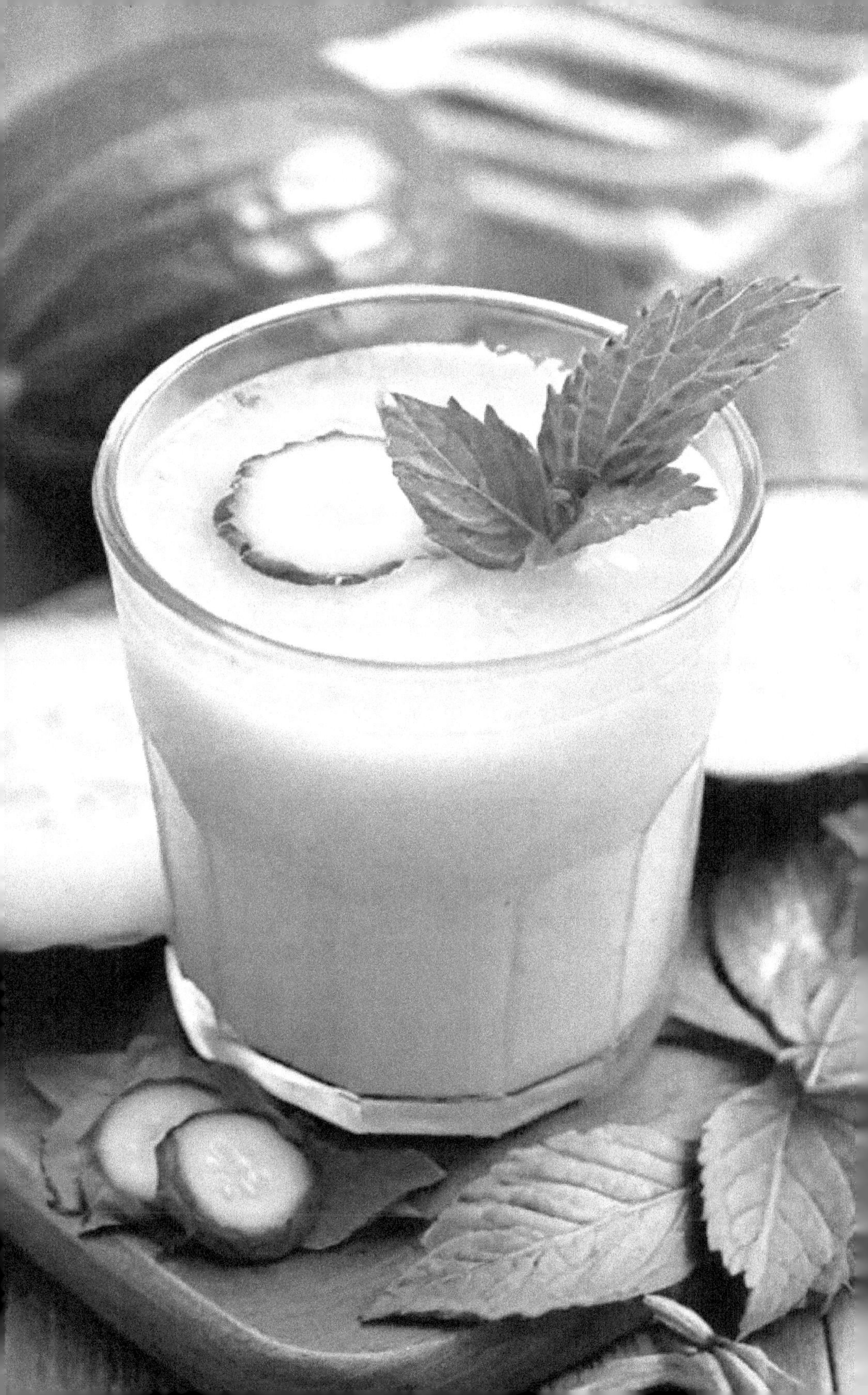

Cantaloupe & Honeydew Juice

This refreshing juice utilizes the potential benefits of cantaloupe and honeydew melons to create a delicious and potentially acid-reflux-friendly beverage.

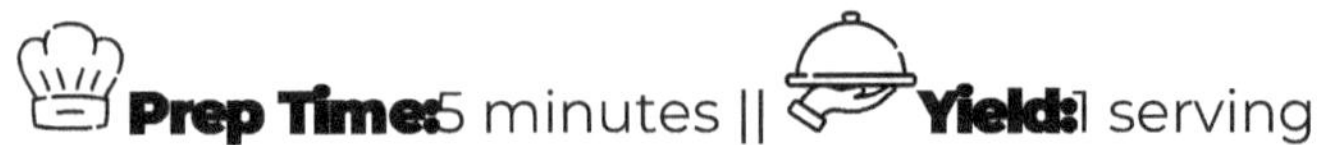
Prep Time: 5 minutes || **Yield:** 1 serving

INGREDIENTS
- 2 cups chopped cantaloupe or honeydew (or a mix of both)

INSTRUCTIONS
1. Wash and chop the melon(s) into pieces that will fit comfortably in your juicer.
2. Juice the melon(s) using a juicer.
3. Enjoy the juice immediately for maximum freshness.

NOTES
- **Cantaloupe & Honeydew Melons:** Both melons are naturally low in acid and high in water content, potentially aiding digestion without triggering reflux in most people. The sweetness can be a delightful alternative to more tart fruits that may irritate your esophagus.

EXTRA TIPS
- Drink this juice on an empty stomach, at least 30 minutes before a meal, for optimal relief.
- Start with a smaller amount of juice, especially if you're not sure how you tolerate melons, to assess tolerance.
- Consider chilling the melon(s) before juicing for an extra refreshing beverage.
- While generally well-tolerated, some people may find melons trigger their reflux. It's always best to listen to your body and adjust accordingly.

Cantaloupe, Honeydew & Mint Juice

This delightful juice combines the potential benefits of melons with the refreshing taste of mint, but use caution with mint for acid reflux.

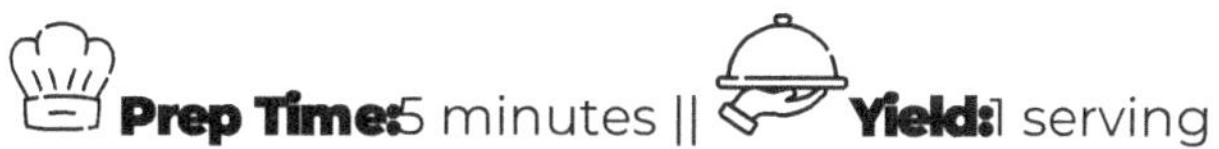

Prep Time: 5 minutes || **Yield:** 1 serving

INGREDIENTS
- 1 cup chopped cantaloupe
- 1 cup chopped honeydew melon
- Sprig of fresh mint (optional)

INSTRUCTIONS
1. Wash and chop the cantaloupe and honeydew melon into pieces that will fit comfortably in your juicer.
2. Wash the mint sprig (optional).
3. Juice the melons and mint (if using) together using a juicer.
4. Enjoy the juice immediately for maximum freshness.

NOTES
- **Cantaloupe & Honeydew Melons:** Both melons are naturally low in acid and high in water content, potentially aiding digestion without triggering reflux in most people. The sweetness can be a delightful alternative to more tart fruits that may irritate your oesophagus.
- **Mint (Use with Caution):** While research is limited, some people find mint aids digestion and provides a refreshing taste. However, peppermint may relax the lower oesophageal sphincter (LES) in some individuals, worsening reflux symptoms.

EXTRA TIPS
- Drink this juice on an empty stomach, at least 30 minutes before a meal, for optimal relief.
- Start with a smaller amount of juice, especially if including mint, to assess your tolerance. Mint can be strong for some people.
- Consider chilling the melons before juicing for an extra refreshing beverage.
- Peppermint may worsen reflux symptoms in some people. If you experience any discomfort after consuming mint, discontinue use.

Soothing Ginger-Turmeric Relief Juice

This simple juice combines the potential benefits of ginger to create a delicious and potentially acid-reflux-friendly beverage.

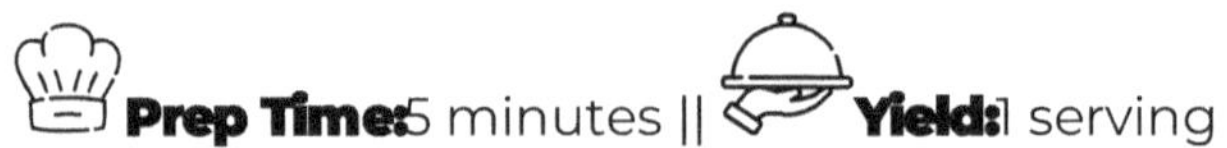

Prep Time: 5 minutes || **Yield:** 1 serving

INGREDIENTS
- 2 cups water
- 1-inch knob of ginger, peeled and chopped
- 1 tablespoon lemon juice (optional)
- Pinch of ground turmeric (optional)
- Honey or maple syrup (optional, use sparingly)

INSTRUCTIONS
1. Wash and chop the ginger.
2. In a saucepan, combine the water and ginger. Bring to a boil, then reduce heat and simmer for 10-15 minutes.
3. Remove from heat and let steep for an additional 5 minutes.
4. Strain the ginger tea into a mug or glass.
5. Stir in lemon juice (optional), turmeric (optional), and a touch of honey or maple syrup (optional) to taste.
6. Enjoy the warm ginger juice for maximum comfort.

NOTES
- **Ginger:** Known for its anti-inflammatory properties, ginger may help reduce reflux discomfort.
- **Lemon Juice (optional):** While citrus fruits can be acidic, a small amount of lemon juice may be tolerated by some and add a refreshing flavor. However, if it irritates your oesophagus, omit it.
- **Turmeric (optional):** Possesses anti-inflammatory properties that may be helpful for some with acid reflux.

EXTRA TIPS
- Drink this warm ginger juice on an empty stomach, at least 30 minutes before a meal, for optimal relief.
- You can adjust the amount of ginger or steeping time to personalize the flavor strength.
- Consider adding a few slices of cucumber (peeled) to the simmering water for extra hydration and a milder flavor.

Tangy Citrus & Ginger Juice

This refreshing juice combines the potential benefits of probiotics and anti-inflammatory ingredients to create a potentially acid-reflux-friendly drink. However, it's important to note that unlike smoothies, juices lack fiber, which can be important for digestion.

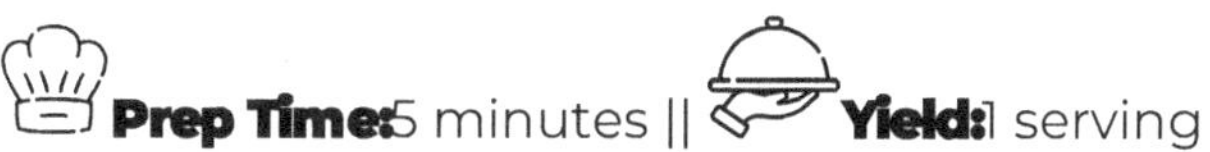

Prep Time: 5 minutes || **Yield:** 1 serving

INGREDIENTS
- 1 cup unsweetened, fresh apple juice
- 1/2 cup fermented kombucha (original or ginger flavour)
- 1/2 inch knob of ginger, peeled and chopped
- 1 tablespoon lemon juice (optional)

INSTRUCTIONS
1. Wash and chop the ginger.
2. Combine all ingredients in a juicer and juice until well combined.
3. Strain the juice to remove any pulp (optional, for a smoother texture).
4. Enjoy the juice immediately for maximum freshness.

NOTES
- **Kombucha:** This fermented tea drink contains probiotics, which may help improve gut health and potentially reduce acid reflux discomfort. Choose unsweetened varieties and start with a small amount to see how you tolerate it.
- **Unsweetened Apple Juice:** A good source of natural sugars for sweetness, but be mindful of portion size as excess sugar can worsen reflux.
- **Ginger:** Known for its anti-inflammatory properties, ginger may help reduce reflux discomfort.
- **Lemon Juice (optional):** While citrus fruits can be acidic, a small amount of lemon juice may be tolerated by some and add a refreshing flavor. However, if it irritates your esophagus, omit it.

EXTRA TIPS
- Drink this juice on an empty stomach, at least 30 minutes before a meal, for optimal relief.

- You can adjust the amount of apple juice or water to dilute the flavor if needed.
- Consider omitting the lemon juice if citrus irritates your reflux.
- Kombucha is a fermented drink and may not be suitable for everyone, especially those with certain health conditions. Consult your doctor before consuming kombucha.
- Juices lack fiber, which can be important for digestion. Consider this when incorporating juices into your diet for acid reflux management.

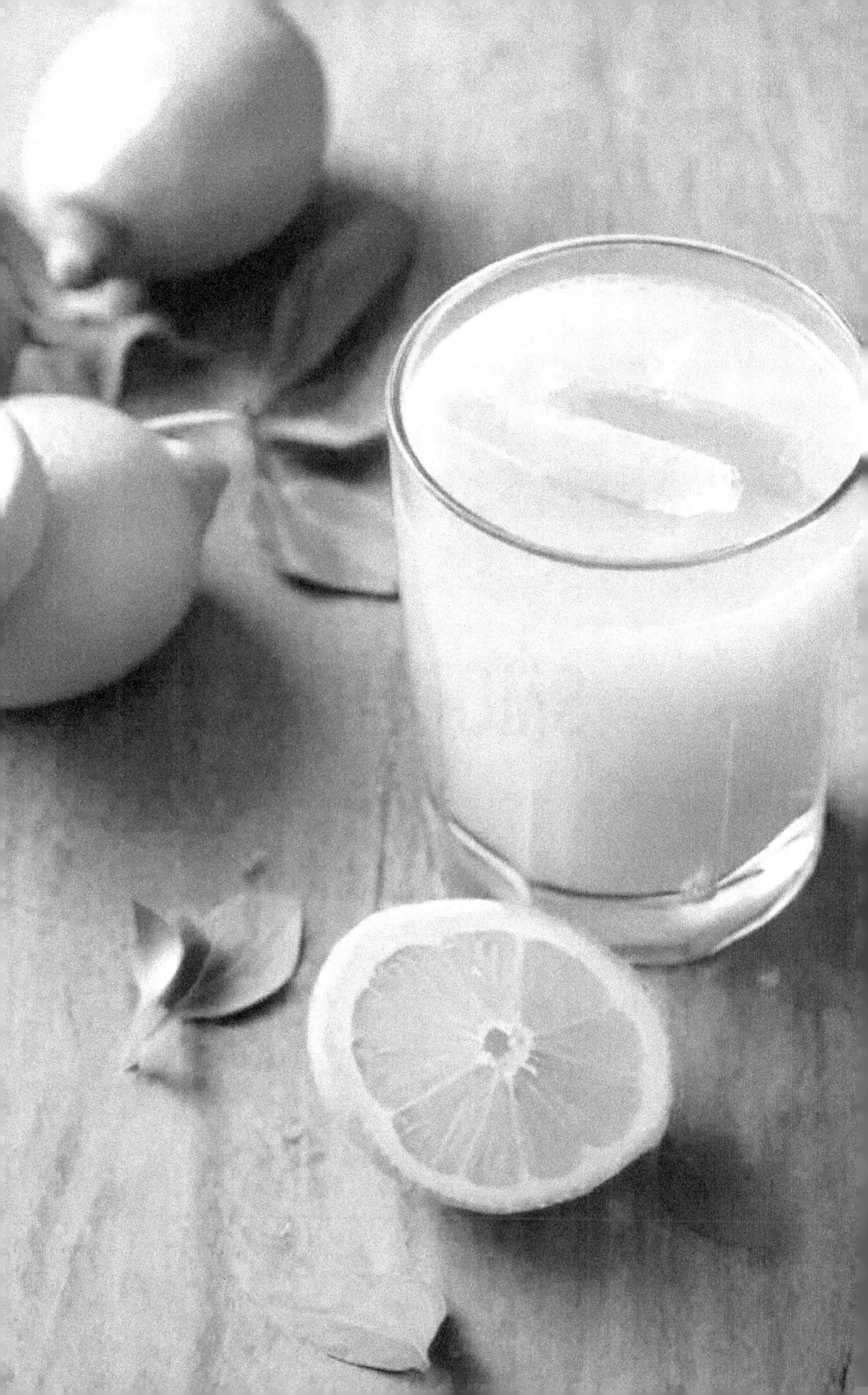

PART TWO

SMOOTHIES

Soothing Papaya & Ginger Smoothie

This creamy and comforting smoothie combines the potential benefits of papaya and ginger to create a delicious and potentially acid-reflux-friendly option.

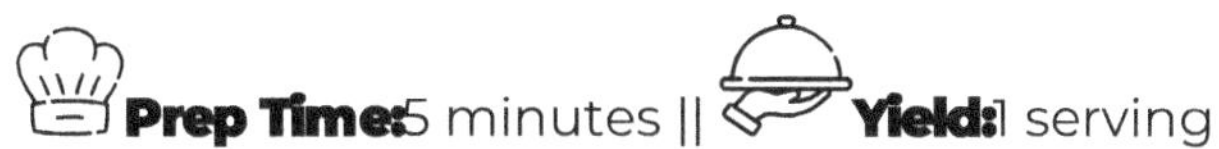

Prep Time: 5 minutes || **Yield:** 1 serving

INGREDIENTS
- 1 cup chopped ripe papaya
- 1/2 inch knob of ginger, peeled and chopped
- 1/2 cup unsweetened plain yogurt (or plant-based alternative)
- 1/4 cup water (or more for desired consistency)
- Ice cubes (optional)

INSTRUCTIONS
1. Wash, peel, and chop the papaya and ginger.
2. Combine all ingredients in a blender and blend until smooth and creamy.
3. Add ice cubes (optional) for a thicker and colder consistency.
4. Enjoy the smoothie immediately.

NOTES
- **Papaya:** Papaya contains an enzyme called papain, which may aid digestion and potentially reduce heartburn.
- **Ginger:** Known for its anti-inflammatory properties, ginger may help reduce reflux discomfort.

EXTRA TIPS
- Drink this smoothie on an empty stomach, at least 30 minutes before a meal, for optimal relief.
- You can adjust the amount of water or plant-based milk to achieve your desired consistency.
- Consider adding a teaspoon of honey or a sprinkle of cinnamon for extra flavor (if tolerated).
- Consult your doctor before consuming large amounts of papaya, especially if you are pregnant or breastfeeding, as it may have laxative effects.

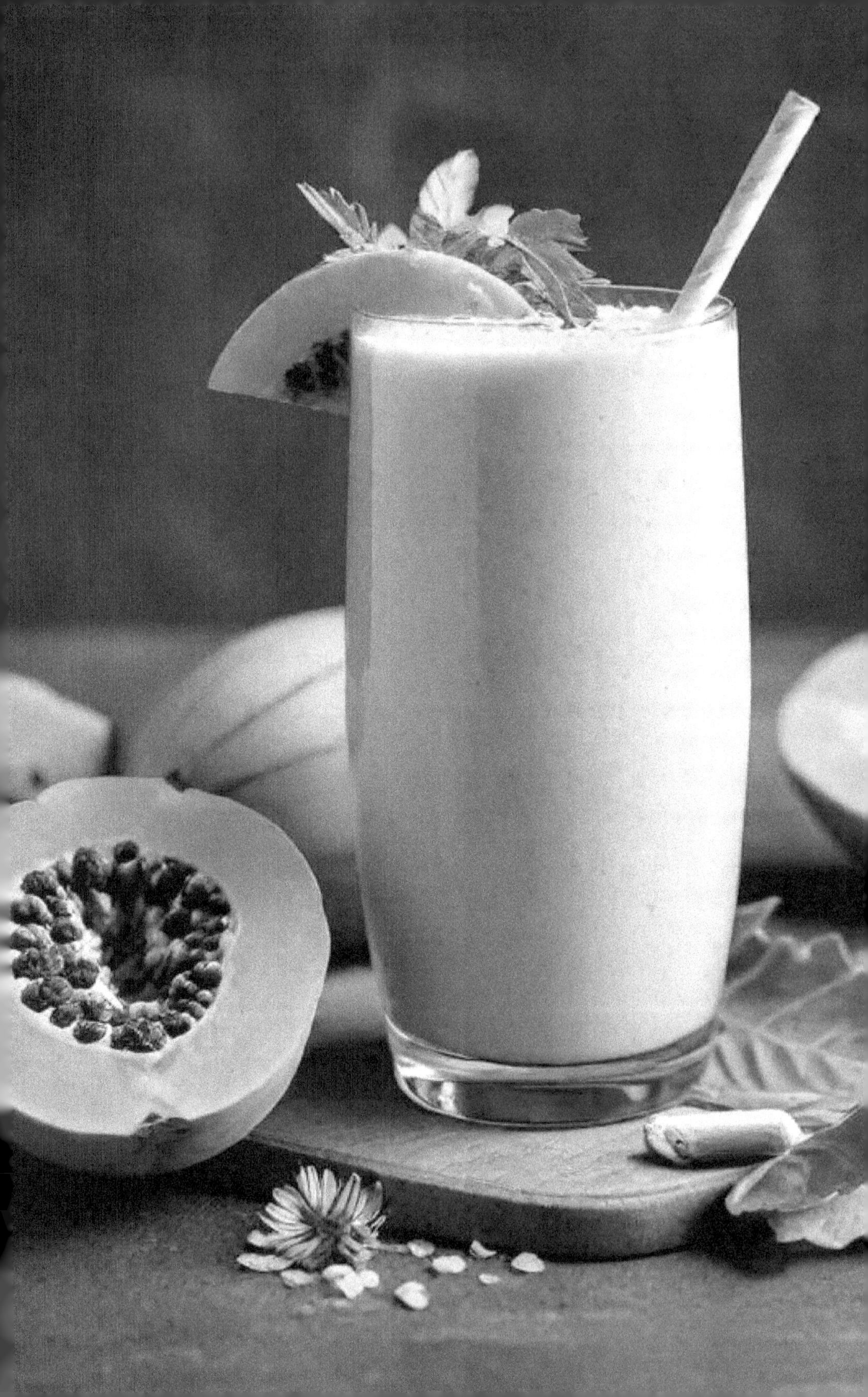

Tropical Oasis Smoothie

This creamy and refreshing smoothie combines the potential benefits of banana and coconut to create a delicious and potentially acid-reflux-friendly beverage.

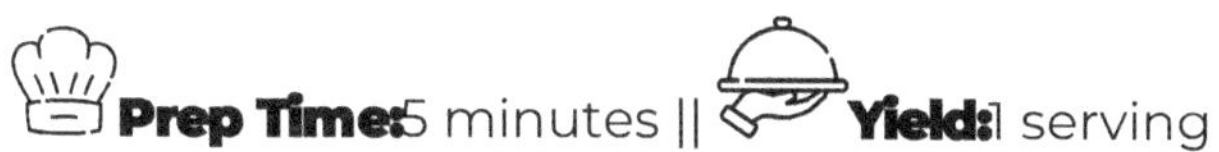

Prep Time: 5 minutes || **Yield:** 1 serving

INGREDIENTS
- 1 ripe banana, peeled and frozen (preferred)
- 1 cup unsweetened coconut water
- 1/2 cup plain yogurt (or plant-based alternative)
- 1 tablespoon chopped almonds or cashews (optional)
- Pinch of ground cinnamon (optional)

INSTRUCTIONS
1. Freeze the banana for at least 2 hours, or overnight for a thicker consistency.
2. Combine all ingredients in a blender and blend until smooth and creamy.
3. Enjoy the smoothie immediately.

NOTES
- **Banana:** Bananas are naturally low in acid and act as a natural antacid, potentially coating the oesophagus and soothing irritation.
- **Coconut Water:** While research is ongoing, some studies suggest coconut water may help with heartburn due to its electrolytes and anti-inflammatory properties.
- **Yogurt (or plant-based alternative):** The probiotics in yogurt may aid digestion and potentially reduce reflux discomfort. Choose plain yogurt or a plant-based alternative with minimal added sugar.

EXTRA TIPS
- Drink this smoothie on an empty stomach, at least 30 minutes before a meal, for optimal relief.
- You can adjust the amount of coconut water or yogurt to achieve your desired consistency.
- Consider adding a handful of spinach (optional) for an extra boost of nutrients.

Summer Delight Smoothie

This refreshing and hydrating smoothie combines the potential benefits of strawberries and watermelon to create a delicious and potentially acid-reflux-friendly beverage.

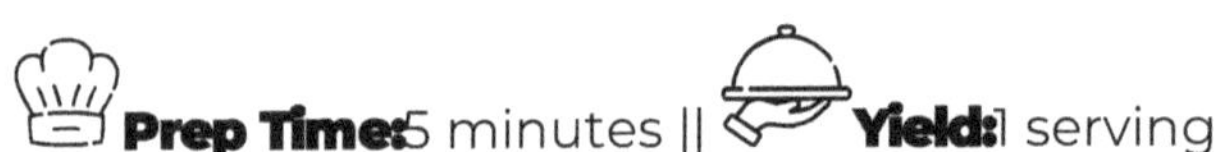

Prep Time: 5 minutes || **Yield:** 1 serving

INGREDIENTS
- 1 cup chopped seedless watermelon
- 1/2 cup frozen strawberries
- 1/2 cup unsweetened almond milk (or plant-based alternative)
- 1 tablespoon chia seeds (optional)

INSTRUCTIONS
1. Wash and chop the watermelon into pieces that will fit comfortably in your blender.
2. Combine all ingredients in a blender and blend until smooth and creamy.
3. Enjoy the smoothie immediately for maximum freshness.

NOTES
- **Watermelon:** Naturally low in acid and high in water content, watermelon helps dilute stomach acid and soothe irritation.
- **Strawberries:** While some berries can be acidic, strawberries are generally well-tolerated by people with acid reflux. They add a touch of sweetness without excessive acidity.
- **Almond Milk (or plant-based alternative):** A good alternative to dairy milk, which can trigger reflux in some people. Choose unsweetened varieties.
- **Chia Seeds (optional):** High in fiber, chia seeds can help with digestion and promote a feeling of fullness, potentially reducing reflux episodes.

EXTRA TIPS
- Drink this smoothie on an empty stomach, at least 30 minutes before a meal, for optimal relief.
- You can adjust the amount of almond milk or water to achieve your desired consistency.
- Consider adding a squeeze of fresh lemon or lime for extra flavor (if tolerated by your acid reflux).

Green Glow Smoothie

This vibrant smoothie combines ingredients that are generally considered alkaline-forming, creating a potentially acid-reflux-friendly beverage.

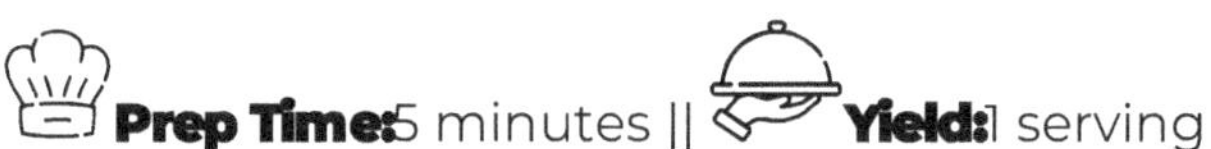

Prep Time: 5 minutes || **Yield:** 1 serving

INGREDIENTS
- 1 cup chopped spinach, washed
- 1/2 banana, peeled and frozen (preferred)
- 1 cup chopped cucumber, peeled
- 1/2 cup unsweetened almond milk (or plant-based alternative)
- 1 inch knob of ginger, peeled and chopped (optional)

INSTRUCTIONS
1. Wash and chop the spinach, cucumber, and ginger (if using).
2. Freeze the banana for at least 2 hours, or overnight for a thicker consistency.
3. Combine all ingredients in a blender and blend until smooth and creamy.
4. Enjoy the smoothie immediately for maximum freshness.

NOTES
- **Spinach:** While research on its direct impact on acid reflux is limited, some studies suggest spinach may aid digestion, potentially relieving acid reflux discomfort. Note: Juicing removes most fiber from spinach, so consider including whole spinach in your diet alongside the smoothie.
- **Banana:** Bananas are naturally low in acid and act as a natural antacid, potentially coating the esophagus and soothing irritation.
- **Cucumber:** Naturally low in acid and high in water content, cucumber helps dilute stomach acid and soothe irritation.
- **Almond Milk (or plant-based alternative):** A good alternative to dairy milk, which can trigger reflux in some people. Choose unsweetened varieties.
- **Ginger (optional):** Known for its anti-inflammatory properties, ginger may help reduce reflux discomfort.

EXTRA TIPS

- Drink this smoothie on an empty stomach, at least 30 minutes before a meal, for optimal relief.
- You can adjust the amount of almond milk or water to achieve your desired consistency.
- Consider adding a squeeze of fresh lemon or lime for extra flavor (if tolerated by your acid reflux).
- Spinach is high in vitamin K, which can interfere with blood thinners. Consult your doctor before consuming spinach if you are taking blood thinners.

Berrylicious Relief Smoothie

This delightful smoothie combines the potential benefits of berries and ginger to create a delicious and potentially acid-reflux-friendly beverage.

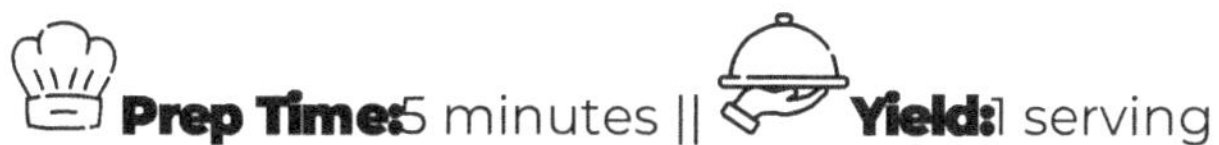

Prep Time: 5 minutes || **Yield:** 1 serving

INGREDIENTS
- 1/2 cup frozen mixed berries (blueberries, raspberries are good options)
- 1/2 banana, peeled and frozen (preferred)
- 1 cup unsweetened almond milk (or plant-based alternative)
- 1/2 inch knob of ginger, peeled and chopped
- 1 tablespoon chia seeds (optional)

INSTRUCTIONS
1. Wash and chop the ginger.
2. Freeze the banana for at least 2 hours, or overnight for a thicker consistency.
3. Combine all ingredients in a blender and blend until smooth and creamy.
4. Enjoy the smoothie immediately for maximum freshness.

NOTES
- **Mixed Berries:** Blueberries and raspberries are generally well-tolerated by people with acid reflux due to their lower acidity compared to other berries. They add a burst of antioxidants and flavour.
- **Banana:** Bananas are naturally low in acid and act as a natural antacid, potentially coating the oesophagus and soothing irritation.
- **Almond Milk (or plant-based alternative):** A good alternative to dairy milk, which can trigger reflux in some people. Choose unsweetened varieties.
- **Ginger:** Known for its anti-inflammatory properties, ginger may help reduce reflux discomfort.
- **Chia Seeds (optional):** High in fiber, chia seeds can help with digestion and promote a feeling of fullness, potentially reducing reflux episodes.

EXTRA TIPS
- Drink this smoothie on an empty stomach, at least 30 minutes before a meal, for optimal relief.

- You can adjust the amount of almond milk or water to achieve your desired consistency.
- Consider using a riper banana for extra sweetness, or adding a teaspoon of honey (if tolerated).
- While blueberries and raspberries are generally well-tolerated, some people may find other berries trigger their reflux. It's always best to listen to your body and adjust the berry mix accordingly.

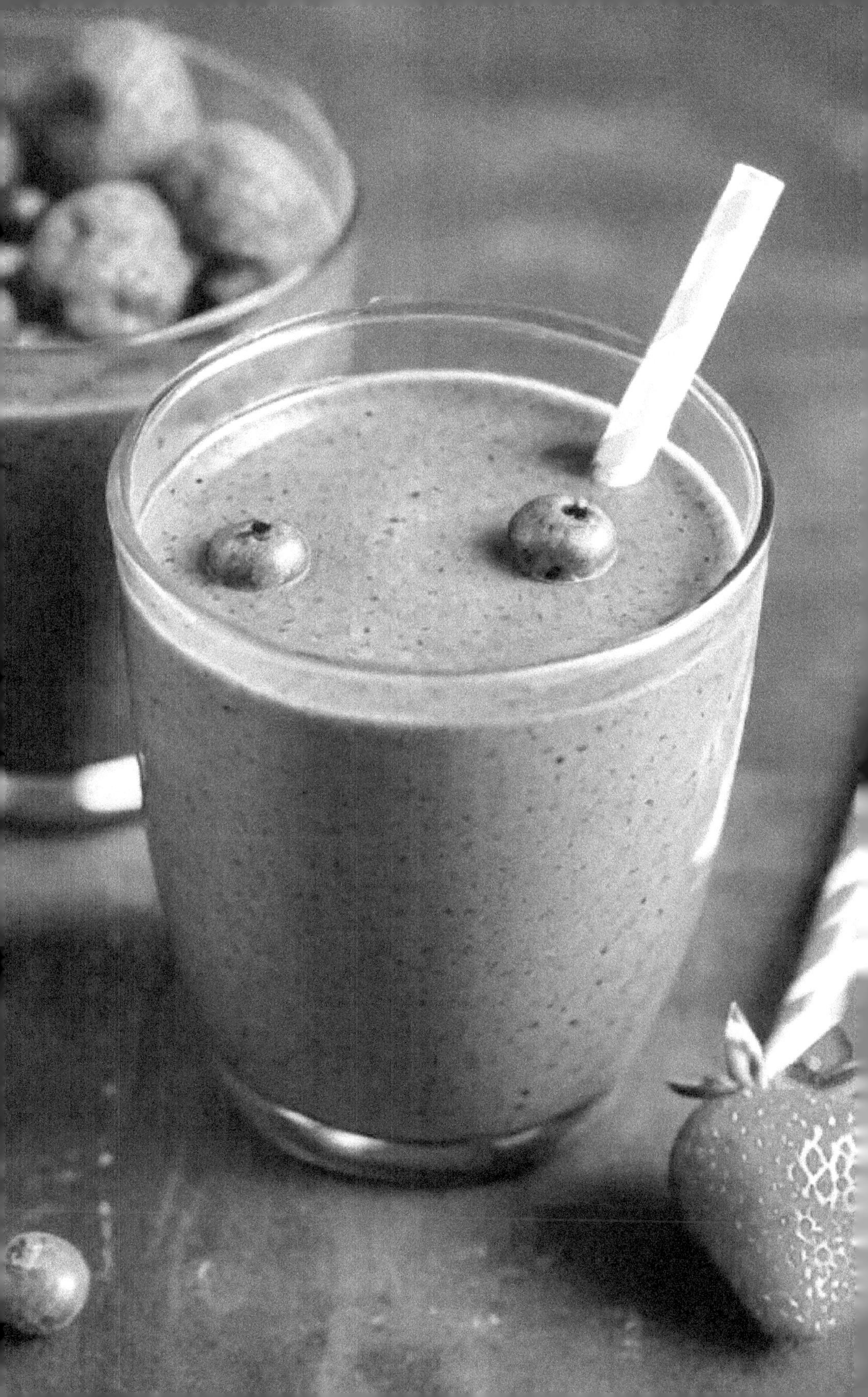

Acai Smoothie Bowl

This vibrant bowl combines the potential benefits of some ingredients for acid reflux relief, but use caution with acai.

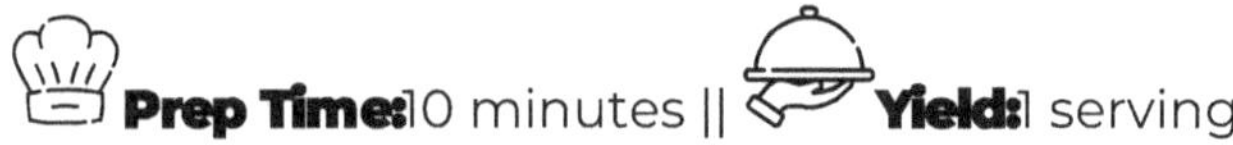
Prep Time: 10 minutes || **Yield:** 1 serving

INGREDIENTS
Base:
- 1 packet frozen acai puree (unsweetened, best to choose a brand without added sugar)   OR - 1/2 cup frozen mixed berries (blueberries, raspberries)

Optional Toppings (Choose Low-Acid Options):
- 1/4 banana, sliced
- 1/4 cup chopped mango
- 1/4 cup chopped pineapple (tart varieties may be irritating)
- 1 tablespoon chopped almonds or granola (optional)
- Sprinkle of chia seeds (optional)
- Drizzle of honey (optional, if tolerated)

INSTRUCTIONS
Using Acai:
1. If using frozen acai puree, let it thaw slightly for easier blending (about 10 minutes).
2. Blend the acai puree with a splash of water or unsweetened plant-based milk until smooth and slightly thick.

Using Berries:
1. Blend the frozen mixed berries with a splash of water or unsweetened plant-based milk until smooth and slightly thick.

Assembly:
1. Pour the blended acai or berry mixture into a bowl.
2. Top with your choice of chopped fruits, nuts, seeds, and a drizzle of honey (if tolerated).

NOTES
- **Acai (Use with Caution):** While some studies suggest acai may have anti-inflammatory properties, research on its impact on acid reflux is

limited. Additionally, many commercially available acai packets are high in added sugar, which can worsen reflux.
- **Berries (Blueberries, Raspberries):** These berries are generally well-tolerated by people with acid reflux due to their lower acidity. They add a burst of antioxidants and flavor.
- **Banana:** Bananas are naturally low in acid and act as a natural antacid, potentially coating the oesophagus and soothing irritation. (Use a smaller portion if using acai due to potential sugar content)
- **Chopped Mango:** Mango is generally well-tolerated by people with acid reflux.
- **Chopped Pineapple (Use Caution):** While some people find pineapple helpful for digestion, its tartness can irritate the oesophagus for others. Consider omitting or using a very small amount.
- **Almonds/Granola (Choose Unsweetened):** Can add healthy fats and fiber, but be mindful of portion size and choose unsweetened options.
- **Chia Seeds:** High in fiber, chia seeds can help with digestion and promote a feeling of fullness, potentially reducing reflux episodes.
- **Honey (Optional, Use in Moderation):** A small amount of honey may be tolerated, but large amounts of sugar can worsen reflux symptoms.

EXTRA TIPS
- If using acai, choose a brand with minimal added sugar.
- Consider using berries as the base for a potentially lower-acid option.
- Enjoy this bowl on an empty stomach, at least 30 minutes before a meal, for optimal relief.
- Start with a smaller portion and adjust toppings based on your tolerance.
- Acai may not be suitable for everyone with acid reflux. It's always best to listen to your body and consult your doctor before consuming acai, especially if you have concerns about added sugar content.

Soothing Sunset Smoothie

This vibrant smoothie combines the potential benefits of papaya, ginger, and oat milk to create a delicious and potentially acid-reflux-friendly beverage.

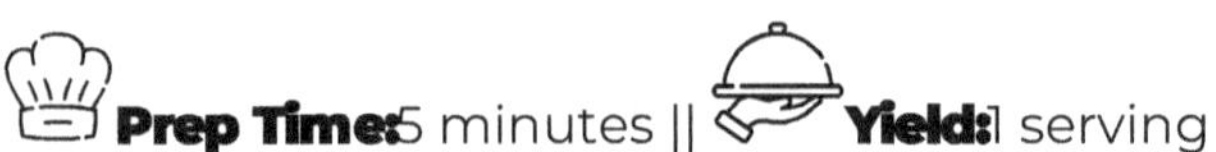

INGREDIENTS
- 1 cup chopped ripe papaya
- 1/2 inch knob of ginger, peeled and chopped
- 1 cup unsweetened oat milk
- 1 teaspoon honey (optional)

INSTRUCTIONS
1. Wash, peel, and chop the papaya and ginger.
2. Combine all ingredients in a blender and blend until smooth and creamy.
3. Enjoy the smoothie immediately for maximum freshness.

NOTES
- **Papaya:** Contains an enzyme called papain, which may aid digestion and potentially reduce heartburn.
- **Ginger:** Known for its anti-inflammatory properties, ginger may help reduce reflux discomfort.
- **Oat Milk:** A good alternative to dairy milk, which can trigger reflux in some people. Oat milk is generally well-tolerated and provides a creamy texture.
- **Honey (optional):** A small amount of honey may be tolerated by some, but it's best to use it sparingly as large amounts of sugar can worsen reflux symptoms.

EXTRA TIPS
- Drink this smoothie on an empty stomach, at least 30 minutes before a meal, for optimal relief.
- You can adjust the amount of oat milk or water to achieve your desired consistency.
- Consider omitting the honey altogether or using a natural sweetener alternative like a few drops of stevia (if tolerated).

Tangy Relief Smoothie

This tangy and refreshing smoothie incorporates ingredients that may promote gut health with probiotics, potentially aiding acid reflux relief.

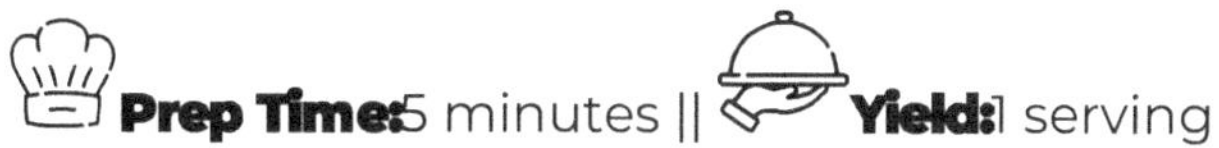

Prep Time: 5 minutes || **Yield:** 1 serving

INGREDIENTS
- 1 cup plain, unsweetened yogurt (with active probiotic cultures)   OR - 1 cup unsweetened plant-based yogurt alternative (with added probiotics)
- 1/2 cup frozen berries (blueberries, raspberries are good options)
- 1/2 banana, peeled and frozen (preferred)
- 1/4 cup chopped mango
- Splash of water or unsweetened plant-based milk (optional)

INSTRUCTIONS
1. Wash and chop the mango (optional).
2. Freeze the banana for at least 2 hours, or overnight for a thicker consistency.
3. Combine all ingredients in a blender and blend until smooth and creamy.
4. Add a splash of water or plant-based milk if needed for desired consistency.
5. Enjoy the smoothie immediately for maximum freshness.

NOTES
- **Probiotic Yogurt (or Plant-Based Alternative):** The live and active cultures in yogurt (or some plant-based alternatives) may help improve gut health and potentially reduce acid reflux discomfort. Choose brands with at least 1 billion CFUs (colony forming units) per serving.
- **Frozen Berries:** Blueberries and raspberries are generally well-tolerated by people with acid reflux due to their lower acidity. They add a burst of antioxidants and flavor.
- **Banana:** Bananas are naturally low in acid and act as a natural antacid, potentially coating the oesophagus and soothing irritation.
- **Mango:** Generally well-tolerated by people with acid reflux, mango adds a touch of sweetness.

EXTRA TIPS

- Drink this smoothie on an empty stomach, at least 30 minutes before a meal, for optimal relief.
- You can adjust the amount of water or plant-based milk to achieve your desired consistency.
- Consider omitting the mango or using a smaller amount if you prefer a less tangy flavor.
- Some people may find yogurt or plant-based alternatives worsen their reflux symptoms. It's always best to listen to your body and adjust accordingly.

Tropical Oasis Smoothie II

This vibrant smoothie combines the potential benefits of probiotics and tropical fruits to create a delicious and potentially acid-reflux-friendly beverage.

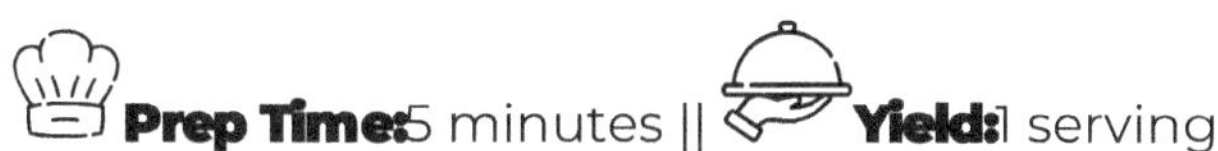

Prep Time: 5 minutes || **Yield:** 1 serving

INGREDIENTS
- 1 cup kefir (unsweetened, plain or flavored)
- 1/2 cup frozen pineapple chunks
- 1/2 banana, peeled and frozen (preferred)
- 1/4 cup chopped papaya
- Splash of water or coconut water (optional)

INSTRUCTIONS
1. Wash and chop the papaya (optional).
2. Freeze the banana for at least 2 hours, or overnight for a thicker consistency.
3. Combine all ingredients in a blender and blend until smooth and creamy.
4. Add a splash of water or coconut water if needed for desired consistency.
5. Enjoy the smoothie immediately for maximum freshness.

NOTES
- **Kefir:** A fermented milk drink rich in probiotics, kefir may help improve gut health and potentially reduce acid reflux discomfort. Choose plain kefir or flavored varieties without added sugar.
- **Frozen Pineapple (Use Caution):** While pineapple can aid digestion for some, its tartness can irritate the esophagus for others. Start with a small amount and see how you tolerate it.
- **Banana:** Bananas are naturally low in acid and act as a natural antacid, potentially coating the esophagus and soothing irritation.
- **Papaya:** Contains an enzyme called papain, which may aid digestion and potentially reduce heartburn.

EXTRA TIPS
- Drink this smoothie on an empty stomach, at least 30 minutes before a meal, for optimal relief.

- You can adjust the amount of water or coconut water to achieve your desired consistency.
- Consider omitting the pineapple or using a smaller amount if you experience discomfort.
- Kefir is a dairy product. If you are lactose intolerant, choose a coconut kefir or another plant-based alternative with added probiotics.
- Some people may find kefir or pineapple worsen their reflux symptoms. It's always best to listen to your body and adjust accordingly.

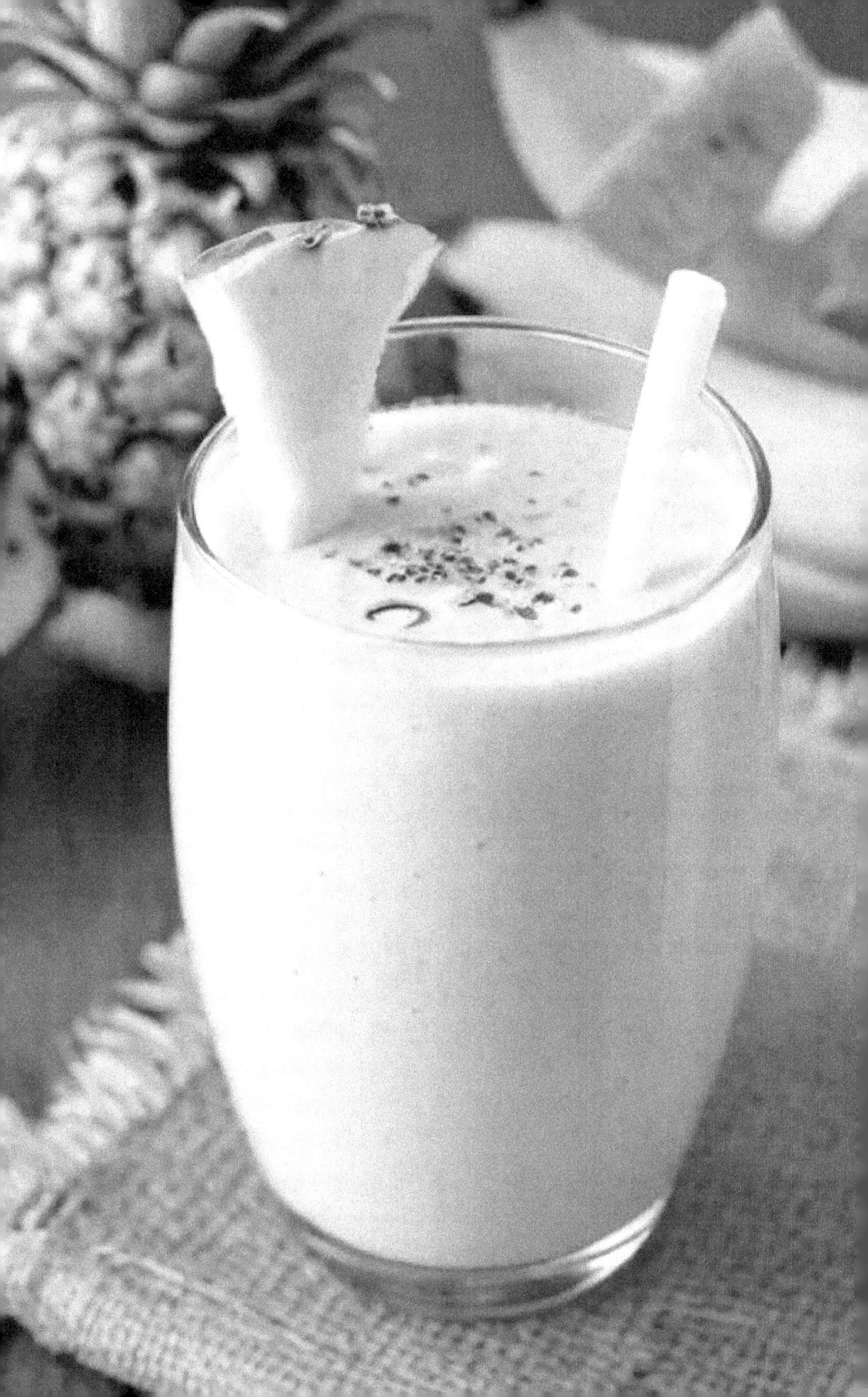

Tropical Twist Juice

This vibrant juice combines the potential benefits of probiotics and tropical fruits to create a delicious and potentially acid-reflux-friendly beverage. However, similar to the previous recipe, juices lack fiber, which is important for digestion.

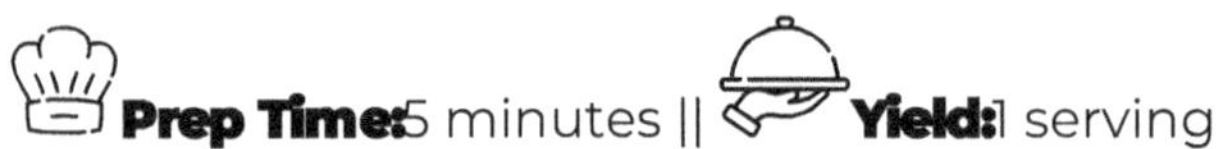

Prep Time: 5 minutes || **Yield:** 1 serving

INGREDIENTS
- 1 cup unsweetened pear juice
- 1/2 cup water kefir (unsweetened, plain or flavoured)
- 1/2 cup chopped pineapple chunks (use caution)
- 1/2 inch knob of ginger, peeled and chopped

INSTRUCTIONS
1. Wash and chop the pineapple and ginger.
2. Combine all ingredients in a juicer and juice until well combined.
3. Strain the juice to remove any pulp (optional, for a smoother texture).
4. Enjoy the juice immediately for maximum freshness.

NOTES
- **Water Kefir:** A fermented water drink rich in probiotics, water kefir may help improve gut health and potentially reduce acid reflux discomfort. Choose plain kefir or flavoured varieties without added sugar.
- **Unsweetened Pear Juice:** A milder and sweeter alternative to apple juice, pear juice offers natural sugars for taste. Be mindful of portion size as excess sugar can worsen reflux.
- **Pineapple (Use Caution):** While pineapple can aid digestion for some, its tartness can irritate the oesophagus for others. Start with a small amount and see how you tolerate it.
- **Ginger:** Known for its anti-inflammatory properties, ginger may help reduce reflux discomfort.

EXTRA TIPS
- Drink this juice on an empty stomach, at least 30 minutes before a meal, for optimal relief.
- You can adjust the amount of pear juice or water to dilute the flavor if needed.

▪ Consider omitting the pineapple or using a smaller amount if you experience discomfort.
▪ Water kefir is a fermented drink and may not be suitable for everyone, especially those with certain health conditions. Consult your doctor before consuming water kefir.
▪ Juices lack fiber, which can be important for digestion. Consider this when incorporating juices into your diet for acid reflux management.

PART THREE

TEA

Chamomile Comfort Tea

Chamomile tea is a popular natural remedy for relaxation and digestive discomfort.

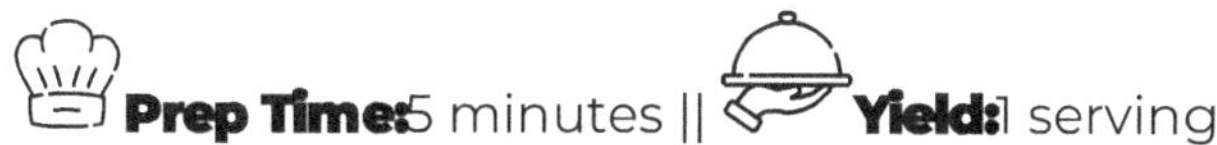
Prep Time: 5 minutes || **Yield:** 1 serving

INGREDIENTS
- 1 cup hot water
- 1-2 teaspoons dried chamomile flowers
- Honey (optional, use sparingly)

INSTRUCTIONS
1. Steep chamomile flowers in hot water for 5-10 minutes.
2. Strain the tea into a mug.
3. Add honey (optional) to taste.
4. Enjoy the warm chamomile tea for relaxation and potential acid reflux relief.

NOTES
- **Chamomile:** Known for its calming properties, chamomile tea may help reduce stress and promote relaxation, which can be beneficial for some people with acid reflux.
- **Honey (optional):** A small amount of honey may soothe a sore throat but use sparingly as excess sugar can worsen reflux symptoms.

EXTRA TIPS
- Drink chamomile tea on an empty stomach, at least 30 minutes before a meal, for optimal relief.
- Consider adding a few slices of ginger (peeled) to the steeping tea for additional potential benefits.
- Everyone's experience with acid reflux is different. While chamomile tea is generally well-tolerated, some people may experience allergic reactions. It's always best to consult your doctor before consuming chamomile, especially if you have any allergies or take medications.

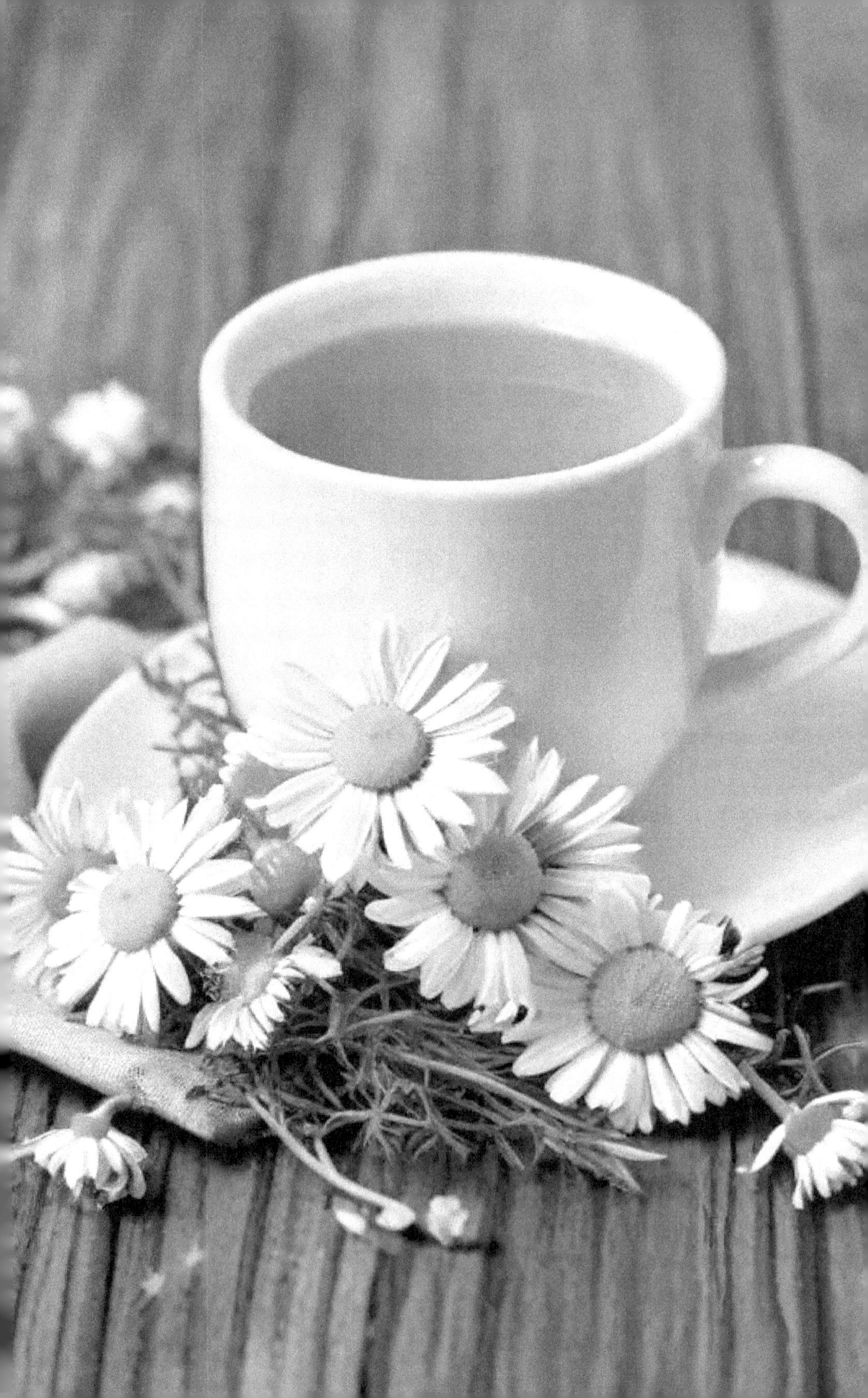

Fennel Tea

Fennel tea is a popular herbal remedy for digestive issues, and it may offer potential benefits for acid reflux. Here's how to make a cup:

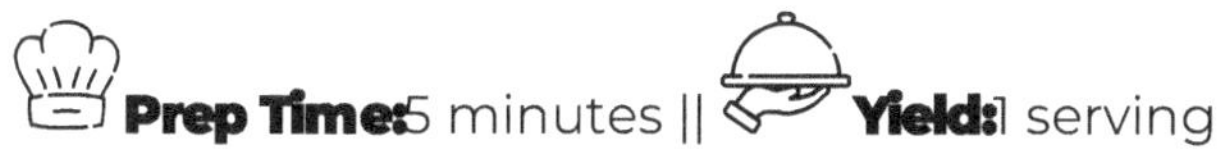

Prep Time: 5 minutes || **Yield:** 1 serving

INGREDIENTS
- 1 cup hot water
- 1-2 teaspoons dried fennel seeds
- Honey (optional, use sparingly)

INSTRUCTIONS
1. Crush the fennel seeds slightly using a mortar and pestle or the back of a spoon (optional). This helps release the flavor and potential benefits.
2. Steep the fennel seeds in hot water for 5-10 minutes.
3. Strain the tea into a mug.
4. Add honey (optional) to taste.
5. Enjoy the warm fennel tea for relaxation and potential acid reflux relief.

NOTES
- **Fennel Seeds:** These seeds contain compounds that may help relax the muscles in the digestive tract, potentially reducing reflux discomfort and gas.
- **Anti-inflammatory Properties:** Fennel may also possess anti-inflammatory properties that can be beneficial for some with acid reflux.

EXTRA TIPS
- Drink fennel tea on an empty stomach, at least 30 minutes before a meal, for optimal relief.
- Consider adding a few slices of ginger (peeled) to the steeping tea for additional potential benefits.
- While fennel tea is generally well-tolerated, some people may experience allergic reactions. It's always best to consult your doctor before consuming fennel, especially if you have any allergies or take medications.

Golden Relief Turmeric Tea

Turmeric tea is a popular beverage with potential benefits for various health concerns, including acid reflux.

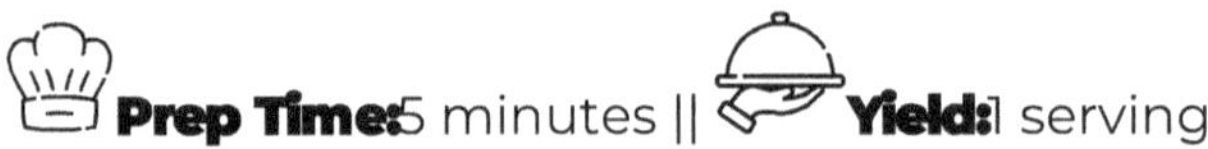

Prep Time: 5 minutes || **Yield:** 1 serving

INGREDIENTS
- 1 cup hot water
- 1 teaspoon ground turmeric
- 1/2 inch knob of ginger, peeled and grated (optional)
- Pinch of black pepper (optional)
- Honey or maple syrup (optional, use sparingly)
- Milk of your choice (optional)

INSTRUCTIONS
1. In a saucepan, combine the water, turmeric, and ginger (if using). Bring to a boil, then reduce heat and simmer for 5-10 minutes.
2. Strain the tea into a mug.
3. Add a pinch of black pepper (optional) to enhance curcumin absorption (the active compound in turmeric).
4. Stir in a touch of honey or maple syrup (optional) for sweetness.
5. Consider adding a splash of milk of your choice (dairy or plant-based) for a creamier texture (if tolerated).
6. Enjoy the warm turmeric tea for relaxation and potential acid reflux relief.

NOTES
- **Turmeric:** This spice contains curcumin, which has anti-inflammatory properties that may be helpful for some with acid reflux.
- **Ginger (optional):** Known for its anti-inflammatory properties, ginger may further reduce reflux discomfort.
- **Black Pepper (optional):** A small pinch of black pepper can significantly enhance curcumin absorption from turmeric.

EXTRA TIPS
- Drink turmeric tea on an empty stomach, at least 30 minutes before a meal, for optimal relief.
- You can adjust the amount of turmeric or steeping time to personalize the flavor strength.

Cardamom Comfort Tea

Cardamom tea is a traditional remedy for digestive issues, and it may offer potential benefits for relieving acid reflux discomfort.

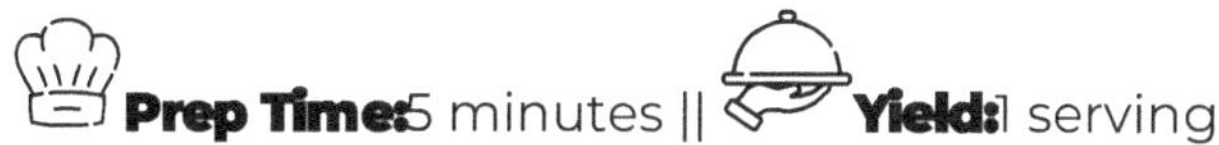

Prep Time: 5 minutes || **Yield:** 1 serving

INGREDIENTS
- 1 cup hot water
- 2-3 cardamom pods, crushed slightly
- Honey (optional, use sparingly)

INSTRUCTIONS
1. Crush the cardamom pods lightly using a mortar and pestle or the back of a spoon. This helps release the flavor and potential benefits.
2. Steep the crushed cardamom pods in hot water for 5-10 minutes.
3. Strain the tea into a mug.
4. Add honey (optional) to taste.
5. Enjoy the warm cardamom tea for relaxation and potential acid reflux relief.

NOTES
- **Cardamom:** This spice has carminative properties, which can help reduce gas and bloating, both of which can worsen acid reflux discomfort.
- **Anti-inflammatory Properties:** Cardamom may also possess anti-inflammatory properties that can be beneficial for some with acid reflux.

EXTRA TIPS
- Drink cardamom tea on an empty stomach, at least 30 minutes before a meal, for optimal relief.
- Consider adding a few slices of ginger (peeled) to the steeping tea for additional potential benefits.
- While cardamom tea is generally well-tolerated, some people may experience allergic reactions. It's always best to consult your doctor before consuming cardamom, especially if you have any allergies or take medications.

Slippery Elm Soothing Tea

Slippery elm tea is a popular natural remedy for throat irritation and digestive discomfort. While research on its effectiveness for acid reflux is limited, some people find it soothing.

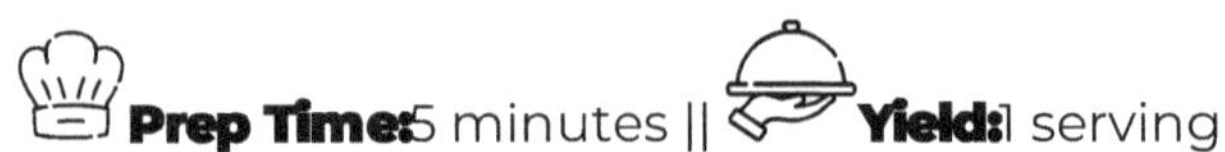
Prep Time: 5 minutes || **Yield:** 1 serving

INGREDIENTS
- 1 cup hot water
- 1-2 teaspoons ground slippery elm bark
- Honey (optional, use sparingly)

INSTRUCTIONS
1. In a mug, whisk together the ground slippery elm bark and a small amount of hot water to create a paste.
2. Slowly whisk in the remaining hot water until well combined.
3. Let the tea steep for 5-10 minutes, allowing the slippery elm to thicken slightly.
4. Strain the tea through a fine-mesh sieve (optional) to remove any remaining bark particles.
5. Add honey (optional) to taste.
6. Enjoy the warm slippery elm tea for a soothing and potentially acid-reflux-relieving beverage.

NOTES
- **Slippery Elm Bark:** Contains mucilage, a gel-like substance that coats and soothes the irritated oesophagus, potentially reducing acid reflux discomfort.
- **Soothing Properties:** The mucilage in slippery elm may also help soothe a sore throat, which can sometimes accompany acid reflux.

EXTRA TIPS
- Drink slippery elm tea on an empty stomach, at least 30 minutes before a meal, for optimal relief.
- Consider adding a few slices of ginger (peeled) to the steeping tea for additional potential benefits.
- **Thick Consistency:** Slippery elm tea can be thick and some may find the texture unpleasant.

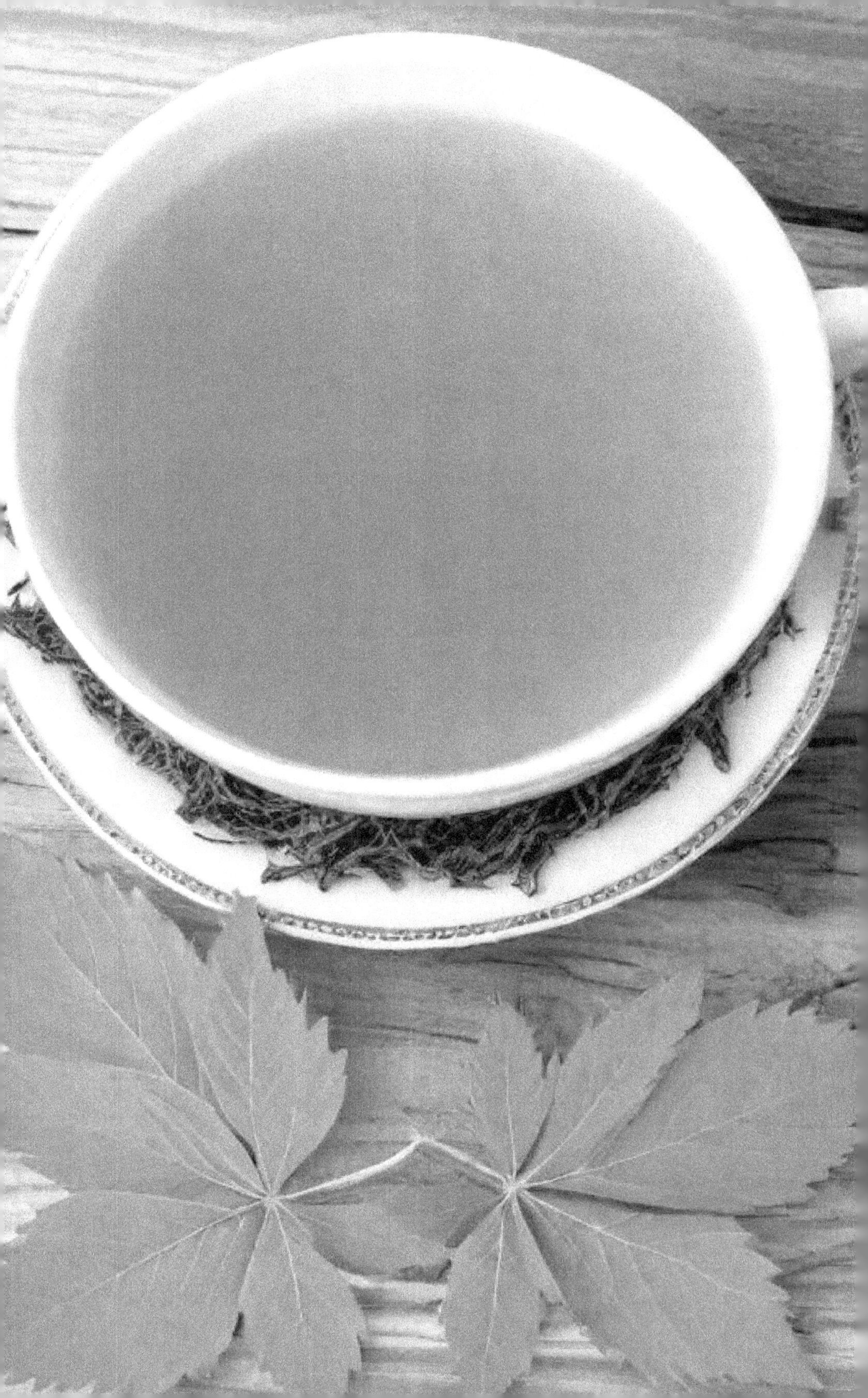

Marshmallow Root Relief Tea

Marshmallow root tea is a traditional herbal remedy used for soothing irritation in the respiratory tract and digestive system. It may offer potential benefits for relieving acid reflux discomfort.

**Prep Time:**5 minutes (cold infusion) or 20 minutes (decoction) || 
Yield:1 serving

INGREDIENTS
- 2-3 tablespoons dried marshmallow root (or marshmallow root powder)
- 1 pint of cold water (for cold infusion)
- OR
- 1 cup hot water (for decoction)

INSTRUCTIONS
Cold Infusion Method (Preferred for Acid Reflux):
1. Measure out the marshmallow root and add it to a jar or container with a lid.
2. Pour cold water over the marshmallow root, making sure all the root is covered.
3. Stir the mixture gently to make sure the marshmallow root is fully submerged.
4. Cover the container with a lid and place it in the refrigerator overnight (at least 8 hours).
5. The next morning, strain the mixture through a fine-mesh strainer or cheesecloth, separating the liquid from the marshmallow root.

Decoction Method (Alternative):
1. In a saucepan, combine the marshmallow root and hot water.
2. Bring the water to a boil, then reduce heat and simmer for 20 minutes.
3. Remove the saucepan from heat and let the tea steep for an additional 10 minutes.
4. Strain the tea through a fine-mesh strainer or cheesecloth.

In Both Methods:
5. You can enjoy the tea warm or chilled.
6. Consider adding a touch of honey or maple syrup for sweetness (use sparingly).

NOTES
- **Marshmallow Root:** Contains mucilage, a gel-like substance that coats and soothes the irritated oesophagus, potentially reducing acid reflux discomfort.

EXTRA TIPS
- Drink marshmallow root tea on an empty stomach, at least 30 minutes before a meal, for optimal relief.
- You can adjust the amount of marshmallow root depending on your desired flavor strength.
- **Cold Infusion Recommended:** The cold infusion method is generally preferred for acid reflux as it helps preserve the beneficial mucilage, which can be degraded by heat (decoction method).

Soothing Ginger Tea

Ginger tea is a popular and well-researched natural remedy for nausea and indigestion, and it may also offer relief for acid reflux.

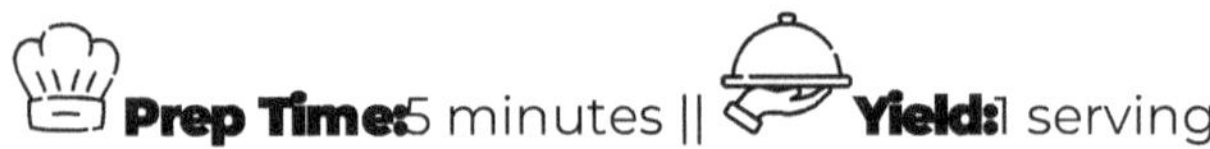

Prep Time: 5 minutes || **Yield:** 1 serving

INGREDIENTS
- 1 cup hot water
- 1-2 inch knob of ginger, peeled and sliced (or 1-2 teaspoons ground ginger)
- Honey (optional, use sparingly)
- Lemon juice (optional, use sparingly)

INSTRUCTIONS
1. If using fresh ginger, slice the peeled knob into thin pieces.
2. In a saucepan or mug, combine the ginger and hot water.
3. Bring the water to a simmer (for fresh ginger) or steep for 5-10 minutes (for both fresh and ground ginger).
4. Remove the saucepan from heat (if using fresh ginger) or strain the tea into a mug (for both methods).
5. Add honey (optional) for sweetness and lemon juice (optional) for a refreshing twist. Remember to use both sparingly as excess sugar and acidity can worsen reflux symptoms.
6. Enjoy the warm ginger tea for a soothing and potentially acid-reflux-relieving beverage.

NOTES
- **Ginger:** Known for its anti-inflammatory properties, ginger may help reduce inflammation in the oesophagus caused by acid reflux.

EXTRA TIPS
- Drink ginger tea on an empty stomach, at least 30 minutes before a meal, for optimal relief.
- You can adjust the amount of ginger or steeping time to personalize the flavor strength.
- Consider adding a few slices of lemon (peeled) to the simmering water for extra hydration and a milder flavor (if tolerated by your esophagus).

PART FOUR

TRACKING JOURNAL TEMPLATE & CONVERSION GUIDE

ACID REFLUX RELIEF JUICE JOURNAL: TRACK YOUR PROGRESS

This journal is designed to help you monitor your acid reflux symptoms and track the effectiveness of your journey with "Acid Reflux Relief Juices Book." By recording your daily experiences and triggers, you'll gain valuable insights and personalize your approach for lasting relief.

Date:

Morning:
→ **Symptoms:** (Note all that apply) No symptoms / Heartburn / Regurgitation / Sour taste / Chest pain / Difficulty swallowing / Other:
____
→ **Severity:** (Rate 1-5, with 1 being mild and 5 severe)
→ **Juice consumed:** (Name of juice)
→ **Breakfast:** (Brief description)

Lunch:
→ **Symptoms:** (Note all that apply) No symptoms / Heartburn / Regurgitation / Sour taste / Chest pain / Difficulty swallowing / Other:
____
→ **Severity:** (Rate 1-5)
→ **Juice consumed:** (Name and recipe number)
→ **Lunch:** (Brief description)

Dinner:
→ **Symptoms:** (Note all that apply) No symptoms / Heartburn / Regurgitation / Sour taste / Chest pain / Difficulty swallowing / Other:
____
→ **Severity:** (Rate 1-10)
→ **Juice consumed:** (Name and recipe number)
→ **Dinner:** (Brief description)

Evening:
→ **Symptoms:** (Note all that apply) No symptoms / Heartburn / Regurgitation / Sour taste / Chest pain / Difficulty swallowing / Other:
____
→ **Severity:** (Rate 1-5)

Additional Notes:
- Record any stressful events or changes in sleep patterns that might influence your symptoms.
- Note any medications you're taking for acid reflux.
- Use this space to track other lifestyle changes you're making, like exercise or dietary adjustments.

Weekly Reflections:
- How do you feel overall this week compared to the previous week?
- Have you noticed any patterns in your symptoms?
- Are there specific juices that seem to be more helpful?
- What adjustments can you make to your routine for next week?

Bonus Section:
- Use this space to record new juice recipes you discover or create.
- Track your sleep quality each night (good, fair, poor).
- Note your daily water intake.

Tips:
- Be honest and consistent in your tracking.
- Use this journal as a tool to communicate with your doctor about your progress.
- Celebrate your successes, no matter how small!

This journal is a valuable companion on your journey to a heartburn-free life. Remember, progress takes time, so be patient and kind to yourself.

KITCHEN CONVERSIONS

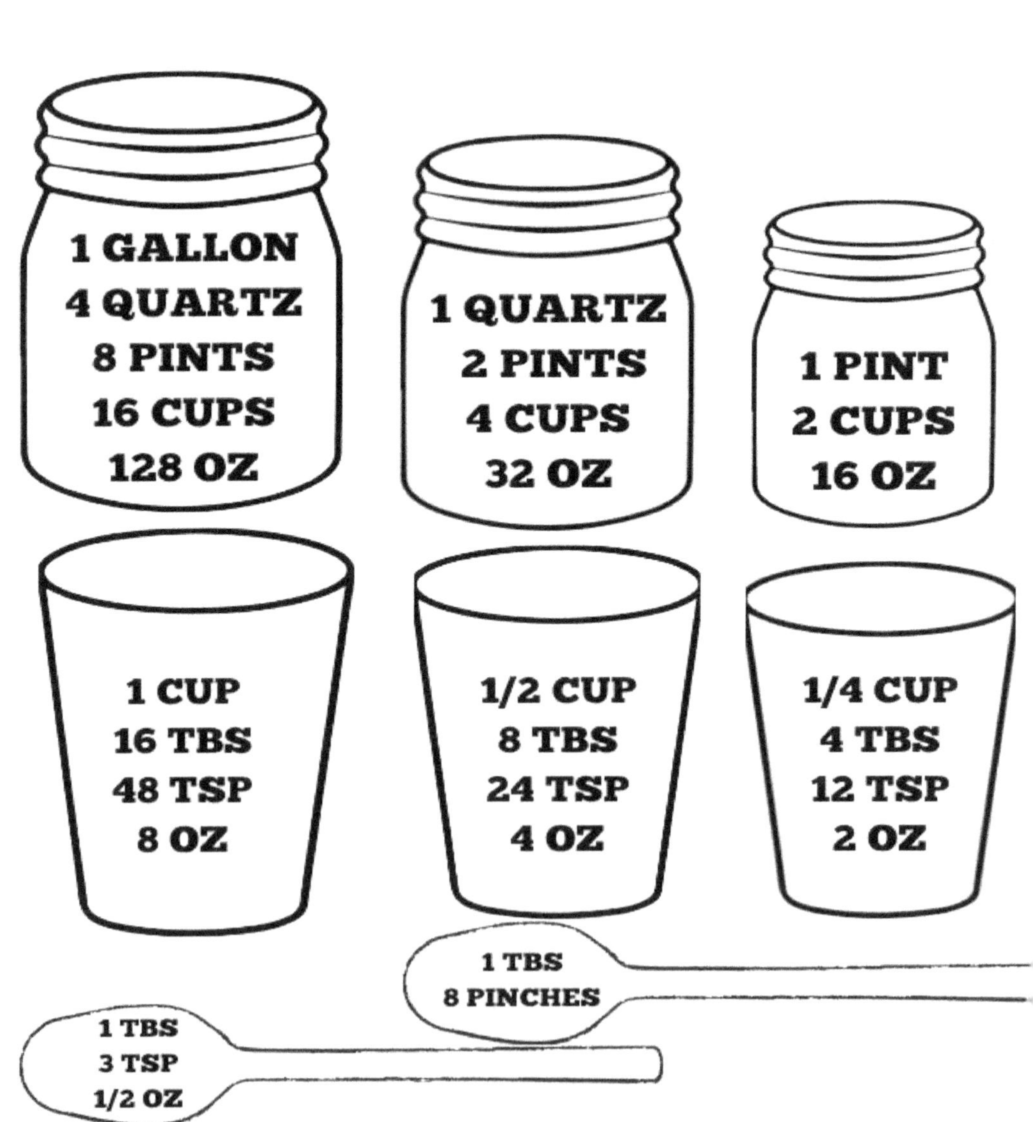

Thank You

Dear Reader,

Thank you for purchasing this cookbook. Creating this cookbook has been a labor of love, and I hope it has inspired you to explore new flavors and techniques in your kitchen. Each recipe has been crafted with care and passion, with the aim to cater to your health and diet requirements.

Your support means the world to me, and I am deeply grateful for your trust in my recipes. As you cook your way through the pages of this book, I hope you find as much joy in making these dishes as I did in creating them.

Jane Garraway

Your Feedback Matters

I would love to hear about your experiences with the recipes in this cookbook. Your honest reviews and feedback are incredibly valuable and help me continue to improve and share the joy of cooking with others. Whether it's a dish that turned out perfectly or one that you think could use some tweaking, your insights are welcomed and appreciated.

Please consider leaving a review on the platform where you purchased this book. Your feedback helps guide future books and ensures that I can continue to provide recipes that resonate with home cooks everywhere.

Thank you once again for your support.

www.ingramcontent.com/pod-product-compliance
Lightning Source LLC
Chambersburg PA
CBHW060751260726
48660CB00002B/568